Lippincott's
Review Series

Fluids and
Electrolytes

Lippincott's Review Series

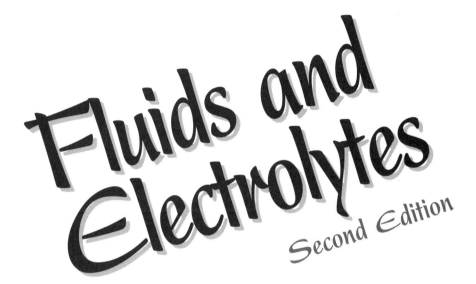

Fluids and Electrolytes

Second Edition

Catherine Paradiso, RN, CCRN, MSN

Senior Manager
Department of Clinical Practice
Meridian Health System
The Medical Center of Ocean County
Ocean County, New Jersey

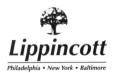

Lippincott

Philadelphia • New York • Baltimore

Acquisitions Editor: Susan M. Glover, RN, MSN
Assistant Editor: Bridget Blatteau
Production Editor: Nicole Walz
Senior Production Manager: Helen Ewan
Production Service/Compositor: Pine Tree Composition, Inc.
Printer/Binder: R.R. Donnelley & Sons Company/Crawfordsville
Cover Printer: Lehigh Press

9 8 7 6 5 4 3 2 1

Library of Congress Cataloging-in-Publication Data

Care has been taken to confirm the accuracy of the information presented and to describe generally accepted practices. However, the authors, editors, and publisher are not responsible for errors or omissions or for any consequences from application of the information in this book and make no warranty, express or implied, with respect to the contents of the publication.

The authors, editors and publisher have exerted every effort to ensure that drug selection and dosage set forth in this text are in accordance with current recommendations and practice at the time of publication. However, in view of ongoing research, changes in government regulations, and the constant flow of information relating to drug therapy and drug reactions, the reader is urged to check the package insrt for each drug for any change in indications and dosage and for added warnings and precautions. This is particularly important when the recommended agent is a new or infrequently employed drug.

Some drugs and medical devices presented in this publication have Food and Drug Administration (FDA) clearance for limited use in restricted research settings. It is the responsibility of the health cre provider to ascertain the FDA status of each drug or device planned for use in their clinical practice.

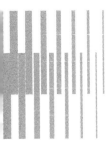

REVIEWER

Charold L. Baer, RN, PhD, FCCM, CCRN
Professor
Acute Care
School of Nursing
Oregon Health Sciences University
Portland, Oregon

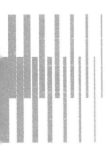

CONTRIBUTING AUTHORS TO THE FIRST EDITION

Angela Curty, RN C, BSN
Nurse Educator
St. Vincent's Medical Center of Richmond
Staten Island, New York
Chapter 12

Patricia Discenza, MSN, RN
Clinical Nurse Specialist
Pediatric Nurse Practitioner
Elizabeth General Hospital
Elizabeth, New Jersey

Pediatric Nurse Practitioner
Department of Adolescent Medicine
Staten Island University Hospital
Staten Island, New York
Chapter 7

Arlene T. Farren, RN, MA
Assistant Professor
Department of Nursing
College of Staten Island
City University of New York
Staten Island, New York
Chapter 11; Test Consultant

Genell Hilton, RN, MS, CCRN, CNRN
Nurse Education Specialist
Critical Care
Beth Israel Medical Center
New York, New York

Adjunct Faculty
School of Nursing
New York University
New York, New York
Chapter 14

Joanne Lavin, RN, EdD
Associate Professor
Kingsborough Community College of the City
University of New York
Brooklyn, New York

Consultant Supervision and Groups
Regents Hospital
Brooklyn, New York
Test Consultant

Donna Marzano-Perrone, RN C, BSN
Nurse Educator
St. Vincent's Medical Center of Richmond
Staten Island, New York
   Chapter 12

Carmen Schmidt, RN C, MSN
Nurse Education Specialist
Beth Israel Medical Center—North Division
New York, New York
   Chapters 2, 3

ACKNOWLEDGMENTS

This book and its companion, *Lippincott's Review Series: Pathophysiology*, were completed through the efforts of a team of people. I would like to thank them all for the dedication, commitment, and zeal they had for these projects. Their work is appreciated beyond words.

Rose Foltz, Developmental Editor. Thank you for devoting so much of your talent, expertise, and, most of all, your time to this project. Also, thank you for your kind and gentle patience. This book was enhanced through your efforts, and it is to the enormous benefit of the readers.

Cheryl Bryant and Karen Spinelli, Manuscript Preparation. Thank you so very much for your commitment, time, patience, and, most of all, *enthusiasm* for these projects. Neither book would have been possible were it not for your work that many times was done in the wee hours of the morning.

David Reuss, Artist. Thank you for sharing your talent with me and the readers of these books. The energy you gave to these projects as well as time and commitment has made this a different kind of book.

Arlene Farren, Test Consultant and Friend. Thank you for saving us in the last days before the deadline. Only a friend in the truest sense could have come through as you did.

Catherine

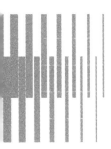

CONTENTS

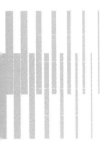

INTRODUCTION

Lippincott's Review Series is designed to help you in your study of the key subject areas in nursing. The series consists of nine books, one in each core nursing subject area:

Community and Home Health Nursing
Critical Care Nursing
Fluids and Electrolytes
Maternal-Newborn Nursing
Medical-Surgical Nursing

Mental Health
  and Psychiatric Nursing
Pathophysiology
Pediatric Nursing
Pharmacology

Each book contains a comprehensive outline content review, chapter study questions and answer keys with rationales for correct and incorrect responses, and a comprehensive examination and answer key with rationales for correct and incorrect responses.

Lippincott's Review Series was planned and developed in response to your requests for outline review books that address each major subject area and also contain a self-test mechanism. These books meet the need for comprehensive subject review books that will also assist you in identifying your strong and weak areas of knowledge. Each book is a complete source for review and self-assessment of a single core subject—all nine together provide an excellent comprehensive review of entry-level nursing.

Each book is all-inclusive of the content addressed in major textbooks. The content outline review uses a consistent nursing process format throughout and addresses nursing care for well and ill clients. Also included are such necessary additional concepts such as growth and development, nutrition, pharmacology, and body structures, functions, and pathophysiology. Special features of each book are Key Concepts and Nursing Alerts, which are identified by distinctive icons. Key Concepts ☼ are basic facts the nurse needs to know to perform his or her job with ease and efficiency. Nursing Alerts ✪ are fundamental guidelines the nurse can follow to ensure safe and effective care.

You can use the books in this series in several different ways. Overall, you can use them as subject reviews to augment general study throughout your basic nursing program and as a review to prepare for the National Council Licensure Examination (NCLEX-RN). How you use each book depends on your individual needs and preferences and on whether you review each chapter systematically or concentrate only on those chapters whose subject areas are particularly problematic or challenging. You may instead choose to use the comprehensive examination as a self-assessment opportunity to evaluate your knowledge base before you review the content outline. Likewise, you can use the study questions for pre- or post-testing after study, followed by the comprehensive examination as a means of evaluating your knowledge and competencies of an entire subject area.

Regardless of how you use the books, one of the strengths of the series is the self-assessment opportunity it offers in addition to guidance in studying and reviewing content. The chapter study questions and comprehensive examination questions have been carefully developed to cover all topics in the outline review.

Unlike the NCLEX examination that tests the cumulative knowledge needed for safe practice by an entry-level nurse, these practice tests systematically evaluate the knowledge base that serves as the building block for the entire nursing educational process. In this way, you can prepare for the NCLEX examination throughout your course of study. Good study habits throughout your educational program are not only the best way to ensure on-going success, but also will prove the most beneficial way to prepare for the licensing examination.

Keep in mind that these books are not intended to replace formal learning. They cannot substitute for textbook reading, discussion with instructors, or class attendance. Every effort has been made to provide accurate and current information, but class attendance and interaction with an instructor will provide invaluable information not found in books. Used correctly, these books will help you increase understanding, improve comprehension, evaluate strengths and weaknesses in areas of knowledge, increase productive study time, and as a result help you improve your grades.

MONEY BACK GUARANTEE—Lippincott's Review Series will help you study more effectively during coursework throughout your educational program, and help you prepare for quizzes and tests, including the NCLEX exam. If you buy and use any of the nine volumes in Lippincott's Review Series and fail the NCLEX exam, simply send us verification of your exam results and your copy of the review book to the address below. We will promptly send you a check for our suggested list price.

Lippincott's Review Series
Marketing Department
Lippincott Williams & Wilkins
227 East Washington Square
Philadelphia, PA 19106-3780

Lippincott's Review Series

Fluids and Electrolytes

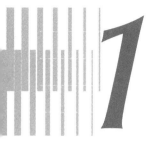

1 Overview of Fluids, Electrolytes, and Acid–Base Balance

I. Basic concepts

A. **Introduction**
  1. A cell and its surrounding environment in any part of the body is primarily composed of fluid (water and solutes).
  2. Interrelated processes maintain balance, or *homeostasis*, within and between the fluid inside and outside the cells.

  3. **Many organs are involved in maintaining homeostasis; these include:**
    a. Lungs
    b. Heart
    c. Pituitary
    d. Adrenal cortex
    e. Parathyroids
    f. Kidneys
    g. Blood vessels
  4. Homeostasis is crucial to sustain life.

    5.   Nursing interventions related to fluid balance are designed to help patients maintain or regain homeostasis, which may be altered by disease.

B.   **Definitions**

    1.   A *solvent* is a liquid that can hold another substance in a solution (water).

    2.   A *solute* is a substance that is either dissolved or suspended in a solution.

    3.   *Body fluid* is a solution of water (solvent) and solutes (electrolytes and non-electrolytes).

    4.   *Electrolytes* are chemical compounds that have an electrical charge (which means they can conduct electricity) when dissolved in a solution. When dissolved in the solution electrolytes are known as ions.:

        a.   *Cations* are positively charged ions.

        b.   *Anions* are negatively charged ions.

    5.   *Nonelectrolytes* are electrically neutral solutes (examples include vitamins, creatinine, proteins, glucose, and lipids); nonelectrolytes that play a role in maintaining fluid balance include protein and glucose.

    6.   *Electrolyte balance* describes the electrically neutral state of the ions dissolved in body fluids. To maintain balance, an equal number of anions and cations must be present on both sides of the cell membrane at all times. A balance of anions and cations must be present for the body's cells to maintain a state of equilibrium.

    7.   A biologic *membrane* is a physical barrier enclosing a fluid space within a living organism (eg, the cell's plasma membrane is the phospholipid-protein bilayer surrounding its contents. The blood vessel wall is another membrane that encloses fluid within a space).

    8.   *Membrane permeability* is the degree to which a membrane allows any substance to pass freely through it.

    9.   *Semipermeable membranes* are selectively permeable, allowing some but not all substances to pass through them.

   10.   *Diffusion* describes the random kinetic motion (known as brownian motion) that causes atoms and molecules to spread out evenly within a confined space until the concentration and distribution are equal in all areas. Diffusion occurs:

        a.   In solutions within completely enclosed spaces

        b.   Through biologic membranes that permit passage of the atoms and molecules from one space to another (eg, from the extracellular space to intracellular space by passing through the cell wall).

   11.   *Filtration* is a physical process in which fluid is pushed through a biologic membrane by unequal pressures exerted by the fluids on either side of the membrane (Fig. 1-1). An example occurs when thinking of a coffee pot. The water pushes the smaller molecules through the filter, leaving the larger ones behind.

   12.   *Osmosis* is the net diffusion of water from one solution through a semipermeable membrane to another solution containing a lower concentration of water and a solute that cannot pass through the membrane.

   13.   *Acids* are substances that can yield hydrogen ions.

   14.   *Bases* (alkalis) are substances that can accept hydrogen ions; these are present as bicarbonate ions.

   15.   *Acid–base balance* refers to a state in which body fluids maintain a stable *ratio* of hydrogen ions to bicarbonate ions.

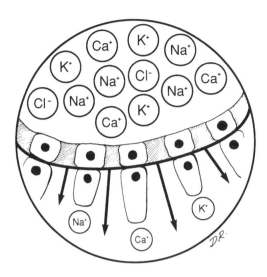

FIGURE 1-1.
Filtration. Microscopic view of glomerular filtration. Fluid (moving along with fluid is
electrolytes) is pushed through small pores in
the filter.

16. The hydrogen ion concentration of a solution, or its degree of acidity or alkalinity, is expressed as *pH:*
    a. Normal blood pH values are between 7.35 and 7.45.
    b. Pure water, a neutral solution, has a pH of 7.
    c. Acidic solutions have a pH below 7.
    d. Alkaline solutions have a pH above 7.
17. *Acidosis* is a condition characterized by an abnormal increase in hydrogen ions or decrease in bicarbonate ions; pH values drop below 7.35.
18. *Alkalosis* is a condition characterized by an abnormal deficit of hydrogen ions or increase in bicarbonate; pH values rise above 7.45.
19. A *buffer* is a substance that regulates pH by maintaining a stable hydrogen ion concentration.

II. Body fluids

A. Function of body fluids
   1. Body fluids:
      a. Facilitate the transport of nutrients, hormones, proteins, and other molecules into cells
      b. Aid in the removal of cellular metabolic waste products
      c. Provide the medium in which cellular metabolism takes place
      d. Regulate body temperature
      e. Provide lubrication of musculoskeletal joints
      f. Act as a component in all body cavities (eg, pericardial fluid, pleural fluid, spinal fluid, peritoneal fluid)

   2. **Water is the principle body fluid and is essential for life. All of the body's processes function best when a person is adequately hydrated. Water is needed for:**
      a. **Digestion**

  b.   Circulation
  c.   Temperature regulation
  d.   Cellular metabolism

B.   **Distribution of body fluids**

1. Total body water (TBW) in an adult equals approximately 60% of total body weight in kilograms (eg, in a 70-kg man, TBW would be 42 kg and would equal 35 L).

2. **Factors affecting the percent of TBW include age and the amount of lean muscle mass versus fat.**

  a.   **Fatty tissue contains less water than muscle.**

  b.   **Older adults tend to lose muscle mass as they age, thereby decreasing the percent of body water.**

  c.   **Infants have a higher percentage (70% to 80%) of body weight as water; this percentage decreases as the child grows older until adult proportions are reached in the teenage years.**

3. TBW is divided among compartments, or spaces, separated by biologic membranes (Fig. 1-2); the two principle compartments are intracellular fluid (within the cell) and extracellular fluid (outside the cell; see Fig. 1-2).

  a.   *Intracellular fluid* (ICF) includes the fluid in all of the body's cells; it accounts for approximately two thirds of TBW (about 23 L in a 70-kg adult). It is separated from the other compartments by the cell membrane.

  b.   *Extracellular fluid* (ECF) includes interstitial fluid and intravascular fluid (plasma) and represents one third of TBW (about 12 L in a 70-kg adult). Interstitial and intravascular fluid compartments are separated by the blood vessel wall.

Total body water (TBW) = Extracellular space + Intracellular fluid space [ICF = ⅔ TBW]

Interstitial fluid space + Intravascular fluid space

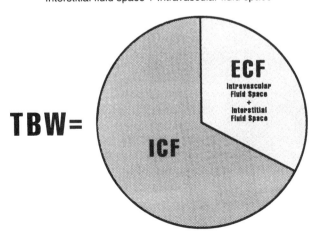

FIGURE 1-2.
Distribution of body fluids.

c. ECF is further divided into 9 L in the interstitial space and 3 L in the intravascular space.

III. Electrolytes

A. Concentration of solutes

1. All body fluid compartments contain water and solutes.
2. The concentration of solutes is in equilibrium among fluid compartments, even though the numbers and types of solutes vary between the fluid spaces.
3. Total solute concentration in body fluids is expressed in *milliosmoles* (mOsm) per liter, a measurement of the number of osmotically capable particles in a given solution.
4. *Osmolality* is a laboratory value defining solute concentration in milliosmoles per liter of solvent; it more accurately reflects the relationship between solute and solvent than the term *osmolarity*, a measurement of the number of solute particles per liter of solution.
5. Osmolarity refers to concentration and dilution:
    a. The more concentrated the solution (or the patient's serum), the higher the osmolarity.
    b. Osmolarity decreases as the solution (or serum) is diluted with water.
6. Because the osmolar concentration of body fluids is very dilute, the difference between osmolality and osmolarity values is negligible. Osmolarity is easier to measure, so it is more commonly used to express the osmotic pressure of body fluids.
7. Osmolarity normally is maintained at 270 to 300 mOsm/L within all body fluid spaces.
8. The concentration of *most* electrolytes in a body fluid is expressed in *milliequivalents* (mEq) per liter, a specific measurement of the total number of that ion per liter.

B. Electrolyte composition of body fluids

1. ICF contains water, electrolytes, proteins, nucleic acids, lipids, and polysaccharides; these cell contents are enclosed by a double-layered, semipermeable membrane.
2. ECF contains water, electrolytes, proteins, red blood cells, white blood cells, and platelets.
3. The primary body electrolytes are sodium, potassium, chloride, calcium, magnesium, phosphorus, hydrogen, and bicarbonate.
4. Major *ICF electrolytes* are potassium and magnesium.
5. Major *ECF electrolytes* are sodium and chloride.
6. **Tables 1-1 and 1-2 illustrate the content of anions and cations in the intracelluar space and plasma. Content of the intracellular space cannot be measured. The plasma content is measured by serum chemistry values. Interstitial content is not measured, but it is essentially the same as the plasma with less proteinate present in the interstitial space.**

TABLE 1-1
Plasma Electrolytes

ELECTROLYTES	mEq/L
Cations:	
Sodium (Na$^+$)	142
Potassium (K$^+$)	5
Calcium (Ca2$^+$)	5
Magnesium (Mg2$^+$)	2
Total cations	154
Anions:	
Chloride (Cl$^-$)	103
Bicarbonate (HCO3$^-$)	26
Phosphate (HPO42$^-$)	2
Sulfate (SO42$^-$)	1
Organic acids	5
Proteinate	17
Total anions	154

(Source: *Metheny, N. (1996). Fluid and electrolyte balance: Nursing considerations, 3rd ed. Philadelphia: Lippincott-Raven page 5, table 1–2).*

C. Tonicity

1. **Tonicity refers to the concentration of particles in solution. It is similar to osmolality.**

2. Body fluids normally remain iso-osmolar to maintain homeostasis; such fluids are called isotonic.

3. Changes may occur in the osmolarity of the fluid in a body space so that its solute concentration makes it either hyperosmolar or hypo-osmolar compared with other body fluids.

 4. A *hypertonic* fluid has a greater relative concentration of solutes, which means that it has a higher concentration of solutes (usually sodium) in solution compared with the serum. A hypertonic solution will pull water toward it to maintain equilibrium.

 5. A *hypotonic* fluid has a lesser relative solute concentration, meaning that the solution is more dilute than the patient's plasma. Water will leave the compartment to maintain equilibrium between compartments.

TABLE 1-2
Approximation of Major Electrolyte Content
in Intracellular Fluid

ELECTROLYTES	mEq/L
Cations:	
Potassium (K$^+$)	150
Magnesium (Mg2$^+$)	40
Socium (Na$^+$)	10
Total cations	200
Anions:	
Phosphate ⎫ Sulfate ⎭	150
Bicarbonate (HCO$_3^-$)	10
Proteinate	40
Total anions	200

(Source: *Metheny, N. (1996). Fluid and electrolyte balance: Nursing considerations, 3rd ed. Philadelphia: Lippincott-Raven page 5, table 1–2).*

IV.   Acid–base balance

A.   Role of acid–base balance

1.   Acids and bases must be balanced to maintain homeostasis in the body's fluids.

 2.   **Homeostasis is crucial for all life processes to occur (eg, cellular metabolism, nerve and muscle conduction, and smooth muscle and cardiac muscle contraction).**

3.   Acid–base imbalances cause changes in the performance of certain body functions such as respirations.

B.   Respiratory regulation

1.   The respiratory system can influence acid–base balance.

2.   Any changes in respiratory rate, rhythm, or depth can result in changes to the balance of acids and bases.

C.   Renal regulation

1.   The renal system affects acid–base balance.

2.   Changes in glomerular or tubular structure and function can alter the kidneys' ability to balance anions and cations.

3.   The renal system will change the way it balances electrolytes to compensate for acid–base imbalances caused by other systems (eg, diabetic ketoacidosis).

Bibliography

Bullock, B. (1996). *Pathophysiology: adaptations and alterations in function* (4th ed.). Philadelphia: Lippincott-Raven.

Drummer, C., Gerzer, R., Heer, M., *et al.* (1992). Effects of an acute saline infusion on fluid and electrolyte metabolism in humans. *American Journal of Physiology,* May, 744–754.

Guyton, A. (1991). *Textbook of medical physiology* (8th ed.). Philadelphia: W. B. Saunders.

Kokko, J., & Tannen, R. (1996). *Fluids and electrolytes* (3rd ed.). Philadelphia: W. B. Saunders.

Metheny, N. (1996). *Fluid and electrolyte balance: Nursing considerations* (3rd ed.) Philadelphia: Lippincott-Raven.

Miller, M.(1997). Fluid and electrolyte homeostasis in the elderly: Physiologic changes of aging and clinical consequences. *Baillieres Clinical Endocrinology and Metabolism,* 11(2), 367–387.

Narrins, R. (Ed). (1994). *Maxwell & Kleemans clinical disorders of fluid and electrolyte metabolism* (5th ed.). New York: McGraw-Hill.

Plante, G. E., Chakir, M., Lehoux, S., & Lortie, M. (1995). Disorders of body fluid balance: A new look into the mechanisms of disease. *Canadian Journal of Cardiology,* 11(9), 788–802.

Porth, C. (1994). *Pathophysiology: Concepts of altered health states* (4th ed.). Philadelphia: J. B. Lippincott.

Rose, B. (1994). *Clinical physiology of acid–base and electrolyte disorders* (4th ed.). New York: McGraw-Hill.

Seaman, S. L. (1995). Renal physiology part II: Fluid and electrolyte regulation. *Neonatal network,* 14(5), 5–11.

Smith, K., & Brain, E. (1991). *Fluids and electrolytes: A conceptual approach* (2nd ed.). New York: Churchill Livingstone.

Szerlip, H., & Goldfarb, S. (1993). *Workshops in fluid and electrolyte disorders.* New York: Churchill Livingstone.

Toto, K. (1994). Endocrine physiology. *Critical Care Nursing Clinics of North America,* December 1994, 647–657.

STUDY QUESTIONS

1. A solute is:
  a. a liquid that can hold another substance
  b. a solution of water
  c. a substance that is either dissolved or suspended in solution
  d. a chemical compound

2. The random kinetic motion that causes atoms and molecules to spread out evenly within a confined space is known as:
  a. diffusion
  b. filtration
  c. osmosis
  d. semipermeable membrane

3. The nurse would analyze an arterial blood pH of 7.48 as indicating:
  a. acidosis
  b. alkalosis
  c. normal pH
  d. inconclusive

4. Which of the following individuals would have the highest percentage of body weight as water?
  a. elderly male
  b. infant
  c. 50-year-old obese female
  d. 45-year-old athletic male

5. Which of the following statements about osmolarity is true?
  a. Osmolarity is normally maintained between 300 and 370 mOsm/L in body fluids.
  b. Osmolarity is a measure of the amount of fluid needed to dissolve solutes.
  c. Osmolarity is a measure of the number of solute particles per liter of solution.

  d. Osmolarity is a measure of the number of electrolytes per solvent.

6. A condition characterized by a deficit of hydrogen ions is termed:
  a. acidosis
  b. alkalosis
  c. isotonic state
  d. homeostasis

7. Which of the following substances regulates pH by maintaining a stable hydrogen ion concentration?
  a. base
  b. buffer
  c. acid
  d. solute

8. When computing total body water (TBW) for a pediatric patient, the nurse is aware that:
  a. Adults have less water as a percentage of body weight than infants.
  b. Infants have less water as a percentage of body weight than adults.
  c. Adults and infants have the same amount of water as a percentage of body weight.
  d. Total body water percentage is determined by genetics.

9. Substances that yield a hydrogen ion are:
  a. acids
  b. bases
  c. cations
  d. anions

10. Hydration of patients is important because water is essential for:
  a. mobility
  b. elimination
  c. circulation
  d. peristalsis

ANSWER KEY

Question	Correct answer	Correct answer rationale	Incorrect answer rationales
1.	c	A solute is a substance that is either dissolved or suspended in solution.	a and b. These responses refer to solvents. d. This response refers to electrolytes.
2.	a	Diffusion (brownian motion) is the random kinetic motion that causes atoms and molecules to spread out evenly within a confined space.	b. Filtration is the process by which fluids are pushed through biologic membranes. c. Osmosis refers to the net diffusion of water through a semipermeable membrane. d. This response is incorrect.
3.	b	Alkalosis is a pH above 7.45.	a. Acidosis is a pH below 7.35. c. Normal pH range is 7.35 to 7.45. d. This response is incorrect.
4.	b	Infants have the highest percentage (70% to 80%) of body weight as water.	a and c. Elderly and obese individuals have a decreased percentage of TBW. d. Total body water in a 45-year-old athletic male would equal about 60% to 80% of total body weight.
5.	c	Osmolarity is a measure of the number of solute particles per liter of solution.	a. Normal range is between 270 to 300 mOsm/L. b. This is a totally incorrect statement. d. There is no measure of the number of electrolytes per solvent.
6.	b	Alkalosis is a condition caused by a deficit of hydrogen ions or an excess of bicarbonate.	a. Acidosis is an increase of hydrogen ions. c. Isotonic describes the number of sodium ions. d. Homeostasis is the state of perfect equilibrium.
7.	b	A buffer is a substance that regulates pH by maintaining a stable hydrogen ion concentration.	a and c. Acids and bases are regulated by buffers. d. A solute is a particle that is dissolved in solution.
8.	a	An infant's percentage of TBW (70% to 80%) is higher than an adult's, making infants more susceptible to complications from fluid losses such as diarrhea.	b, c, and d. These responses are incorrect as they relate to total body water.

Question	Correct answer	Correct answer rationale	Incorrect answer rationales
9.	a	Acids are substances that yield hydrogen ions.	b. Bases are substances that accept hydrogen ions. c. Cations are positively charged ions. d. Anions are negatively charged ions.
10.	c	Water is essential for circulation. This process allows for oxygen to be delivered, carbon dioxide to be eliminated, and all essential elements to be transported to the body's organs.	a, b, d. All of these functions are improved with adequate hydration. Circulation is the *best* answer.

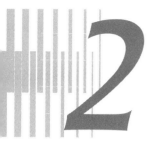

Body Fluid Balance

I. **Sources of fluid intake and loss**

A. **Normal sources of fluid intake**

1. A healthy adult ingests fluids as part of normal dietary intake.
2. Ingested fluids and water in foods account for 90% of daily fluid intake, or approximately 2500 mL.
3. Approximately 10% of daily fluid intake (about 200–300 mL) results from by-products of cellular metabolism (eg, water from oxidation).

B. **Normal fluid loss**

1. Daily fluid balance is maintained because the lungs, skin, gastrointestinal (GI) tract, and kidneys excrete varying amounts of water equal to the total volume ingested.
2. *Insensible* water loss is not visible or measurable and occurs through evaporation and respiration. Approximately 500 mL of water in the form of exhaled vapor is lost through respiration.
3. *Sensible* water loss is visible or measurable and occurs in the form of urine, sweat, and feces:

a. The kidneys excrete water in urine, approximately 800 to 1500 mL/d.

b. The skin loses approximately 500 to 600 mL of water through perspiration and evaporation; this amount can vary widely depending on the ambient temperature and the presence of fever.

c. Because most of the water produced by the GI tract is reabsorbed, water lost in feces accounts for only approximately 100 to 200 mL of the daily total.

4. Because daily urinary output is roughly equivalent to the amount of free fluid intake, an individual's water balance can be estimated by comparing oral liquid intake to urine output. (The other routes of water loss generally cancel out the water taken in through food and cellular metabolism.)

C. Abnormal sources of fluid intake

1. **Abnormal sources of fluid intake include:**
    a. **Intravenous (IV) solutions**
    b. **Total parenteral nutrition (TPN)**
    c. **Blood volume replacements**
    d. **Colloids**

2. IV solutions containing fluids and electrolytes (eg, crystalloids) are used to replace volume and correct abnormalities.

3. TPN, an IV fluid providing concentrated glucose, protein, electrolytes, trace elements, and lipids, is used for patients who are unable to take in food or fluids through the digestive tract.

4. Whole blood, packed red blood cells, or plasma are used to replace blood volume that may have been lost through disease, trauma, or surgery.

5. Colloids (eg, albumin or dextran) are used for replacement or to manipulate fluid shifts among compartments in disease states.

6. Figure 2-1 illustrates abnormal sources of fluid intake.

7. **The nurse should always be concerned that the intake of fluid is being regulated externally to the patient. The patient must be able to circulate the volume of fluid administered to avoid complications such as congestive heart failure.**

D. Abnormal fluid loss

1. **Abnormal fluid loss occurs secondary to:**
    a. **Disease-related processes**
    b. **Trauma**
    c. **Medical interventions**

2. Disease-related processes that result in abnormal fluid loss include:
    a. Vomiting
    b. Diarrhea
    c. Diuresis
    d. Diaphoresis

3. Excessive fluid also can be lost if a person is breathing or perspiring at an increased rate for a prolonged time.

4. Trauma can result in whole blood loss (eg, bleeding or hemorrhage) and serum loss (eg, burns or mechanical debridement of skin).

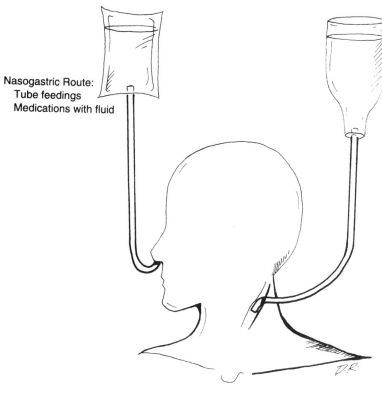

Nasogastric Route:
 Tube feedings
 Medications with fluid

Parenteral Route:
 IV solutions
 TPN
 Blood products
 Colloids

FIGURE 2-1.
Abnormal sources of fluid intake.

5. Medical interventions that may cause abnormal fluid loss include:
   a. Prescribing of certain medications (eg, diuretics that increase urine output and antibiotics that have the side effect of diarrhea)
   b. Treatments such as phlebotomy (which removes blood) or nasogastric and intestinal intubation with gastrointestinal decompression through suction (which removes GI fluids and electrolytes)
   c. Surgical procedures such as small bowel resection with ileostomy, which diverts GI contents outside the body before normal fluid reabsorption occurs in the large intestine
   d. Insertion of surgical drains
6. Figure 2-2 provides more information about abnormal fluid loss.
7. **Abnormal fluid loss is always a concern because the loss cannot always be controlled and a patient can rapidly become compromised.**

II. Dynamics of fluid balance

A. **Complexity**
   1. Fluids must be balanced throughout all of the body's compartments.

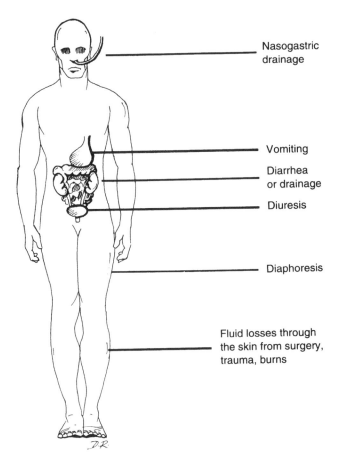

FIGURE 2-2.
Abnormal routes of fluid loss.

2.   Influencing the balance of fluids is:
   a.   The heart (the force of cardiac contractions is significant for fluid balance)
   b.   Blood vessels (vasodilation and vasoconstriction influences balance)
   c.   Endocrine and renal system (hormones and electrolytes)
   d.   Respiratory system (hypoventilation and hyperventilation influences loss carbon dioxide and water, which effects fluid and electrolytes)
   e.   Gastrointestinal tract (where fluids and electrolytes are absorbed and eliminated)
   f.   The size of the body's compartment.

   B.   Location: Body fluids are found in the heart (pericardial sac), lungs (pleural fluid), nervous system (spinal fluid), eye (aqueous humor), musculoskeletal system (synovial fluid), abdominal wall (peritoneal space), gastrointestinal system (saliva, gastric and intestinal fluids).

C. Passive transport

1. Passive transport mechanisms do not involve the expenditure of cellular energy to move water (and the molecules and particles dissolved and suspended in it) back and forth across biologic membranes and between fluid spaces. These mechanisms include:
   a. Osmosis
   b. Diffusion
2. Distribution of body fluid among compartments is maintained by two opposing properties exerted by solutions contained within confined spaces. These properties are:
   a. *Osmotic pressure:* Pressure exerted on a semipermeable membrane; fluids moving from an area of higher concentration to one of lower concentration until equilibrium is achieved
   b. *Hydrostatic pressure:* Pressure of a fluid mass pushing outward against the boundaries of its container (eg, the heart pumps blood, which exerts pressure on the blood vessel wall causing pulsations against the blood vessel walls, known as the pulse).
3. The osmotic pressure and hydrostatic pressure oppose each other within the confines of the fluid compartments to maintain equilibrium. These opposing forces are illustrated in Figure 2-3 which also illustrates capillary dynamics.
4. The presence of a concentration of solute (eg, sodium) draws a solvent (water) through a selectively permeable membrane when the solute cannot diffuse through the membrane. *Osmosis* occurs when there is a *pressure* gradient—a higher concentration of water in solution on one side of the membrane than the other. Fluid moves "downhill."
5. In *diffusion,* the solute moves from an area of higher concentration to one of lower concentration (downhill).
6. When the boundaries of the container are a biologic membrane, the fluid will be pushed through the membrane if there is a pressure gradient—a sit-

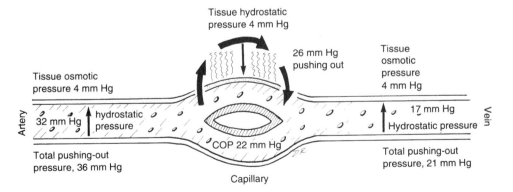

FIGURE 2-3.
Capillary dynamics illustrating pressures at arterial and venous ends.

uation in which the hydrostatic pressure is greater in one space than in another.

7. Fluid achieves equilibrium by moving downhill from the space with the higher hydrostatic pressure and across the membrane to the space with the lower hydrostatic pressure. When water moves through a semipermeable membrane, smaller weight molecules (such as electrolytes) will move along with the water. Larger weight molecules (such as red blood cells, white blood cells, proteins) will remain on the other side of the membrane. This process is called *filtration*.

8. The physical processes that aid in fluid exchange at the intravascular–interstitial level are collectively called capillary dynamics, or Starling's law.

9. Capillaries are the single-cell thickness interface between the fluids in the intravascular space and the interstitial space.

10. Capillary dynamics are directly related to the hydrostatic pressure differences between the venous and arterial ends of the capillary.

11. Water, electrolytes, and cell nutrients are *pushed from* the arterial end of the capillary outward by the pumping action of the heart (hydrostatic pressure) through the capillary cell wall membrane.

12. **At the same time, water, cellular waste products, and electrolytes are *pulled into* the venous end of the capillary by osmotic pressures created by the magnetic properties of plasma proteins.**

13. **Plasma proteins include (in order of abundance):**
    a. **Albumin: Maintains colloidal osmotic pressure inside the extracellular fluid (ECF) and cell wall integrity**
    b. **Globulins: Responsible for immune functioning**
    c. **Fibrinogen: Responsible for blood clotting**

14. Proteins play a role in the dynamics of fluid balance by keeping fluid inside the cell (through maintenance of the normal cell membrane) and by keeping fluid in the extracellular space (through maintenance of blood vessel integrity).

15. The hydrostatic pressure generated by the pumping action of the heart is 32 mm Hg at the arterial end of the capillary, while the osmotic pressure in the interstitial space is 4 mm Hg, for a total of 36 mm Hg outward pushing pressure.

16. Within the capillary, plasma proteins (primarily albumin) maintain a stable colloidal osmotic pressure of 22 mm Hg; these plasma proteins are not permeable through the capillary cell wall, as are dissolved substances such as electrolytes.

17. The colloidal osmotic pressure combined with the tissue hydrostatic pressure of 4 mm Hg equals 26 mm Hg; the net 10 mm Hg difference (36 – 26 mm Hg) is the force *pushing out* fluid from the plasma volume.

18. Plasma hydrostatic pressure gradually decreases (due to less volume and greater distance from the heart) to 17 mm Hg at the venous end of the capillary, while the tissue osmotic pressure remains constant at 4 mm Hg (Fig. 2-3).

19. The total outward pushing force at the venous end of the capillary becomes only 21 mm Hg. At the same time, interstitial hydrostatic pressure, which has increased slightly to 6 mm Hg, adds to the unchanged colloidal os-

motic pressure (22 mm Hg) and creates a total pressure of 28 mm Hg *pulling back* fluid into the plasma volume.

20. The net force drawing fluid into the plasma volume at the capillary venous end is 7 mm Hg (28 − 21 mm Hg).

21. Fluid lost from the plasma to the interstitial space (due to the greater pushing out pressure versus drawing in pressure) is returned to the circulation by the lymphatic system, maintaining normal blood volume.

22. Facilitated diffusion is a specialized type of passive transport requiring the participation of a carrier protein for some substances to cross semipermeable membranes. It is the mechanism by which glucose and most amino acids are able to diffuse into or out of cells.

D. **Active transport**

1. Active transport occurs when dissolved or suspended substances cross cell membranes, requiring the expenditure of cellular energy.

2. Active transport processes or "pumps" are fueled by the cellular energy released when adenosine triphosphate molecules are split (Fig. 2-4); this energy release permits "uphill" movement of substances (movement against pressure or concentration gradients).

3. Active transport can move different substances into and out of a cell simultaneously.

4. The best known example of active transport is the *sodium-potassium pump,* in which sodium ions are pumped *into* and potassium ions are pumped *out* of a cell during each exchange. Other electrolytes also are pumped into and out of the cell (Fig. 2-5).

5. The sodium-potassium pump plays a key role in the maintenance of intracellular fluid (ICF) volume. The outflow of sodium ions counterbalances the osmotic pressure exerted by the intracellular proteins to pull excess water into cells.

III.   **Regulation of body fluids**

A. **Overview of systemic regulators**

1. To maintain homeostasis, many body systems interact to ensure a balance of fluid intake and output and a normal distribution of body fluids among compartments.

2. The primary systemic regulators of body fluid are:
    a. **Renal**
    b. **Endocrine**
    c. **Cardiovascular**
    d. **Gastrointestinal**
    e. **Pulmonary**

3. **The nurse must be aware that disorders in these organs leave a person at a high risk to develop problems with fluid and electrolyte balance.**

B. **Renal regulation**

1. **The kidneys are the major regulators of sodium and water balance in the ECF (Fig. 2-6).**

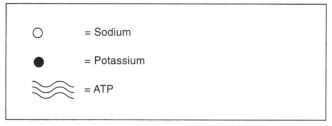

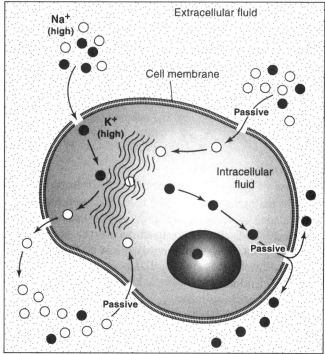

FIGURE 2-4.
Active transport. Sodium that diffuses into the cell through a pore in the cell membrane is actively pumped out of the cell by a carrier system (wavy lines). Similarly, potassium that diffuses out of the cell is actively replaced by the carrier system.

2. Cells in the glomerulus secrete the enzyme renin when they sense decreased serum sodium concentration or decreased plasma volume.
3. Renin activates angiotensin I, which is then enzymatically converted to angiotensin II, a powerful vasoconstrictor.
4. Angiotensin II selectively constricts portions of the arteriole in the nephron. If serum sodium is low in the presence of increased plasma volume, glomerular filtration is increased, thus increasing urine output. If serum sodium is high with normal to low plasma volume, glomerular filtration is decreased, thus decreasing urine output.

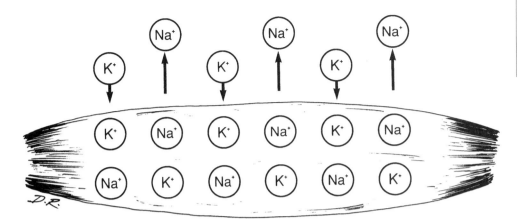

FIGURE 2-5.
Sodium-potassium pump. Sodium ions are pumped into the cell and potassium ions are pumped out of the cell.

  5. Angiotensin II also causes release of the hormone aldosterone from the adrenal cortex; it acts on the distal renal tubule to cause reabsorption of sodium and water and excretion of potassium (Fig. 2-7).

  C. Endocrine regulation

  1. **The primary regulator of water intake is the thirst center in the hypothalamus.**

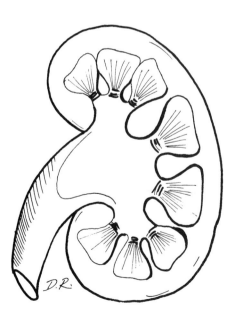

FIGURE 2-6.
The kidney. The kidney regulates body fluids and electrolytes by eliminating water and waste products, and by balancing electrolytes, acids, and bases.

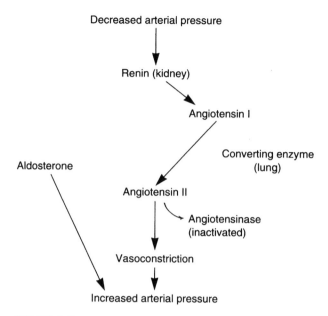

FIGURE 2-7.
Renin-angiotensin-aldosterone mechanism.

   2.   A person drinks or stops drinking water or other fluids in response to a feedback loop of signals from the thirst center and the GI tract. Decreased ICF in thirst center cells, plus decreased fullness in the gut, stimulates drinking.

   3.   Osmoreceptor cells in the posterior hypothalamus respond to changes in ECF osmolarity:

      a.   When ECF osmolarity increases, the pituitary gland secretes antidiuretic hormone (ADH).

      b.   When ECF osmolarity decreases, ADH secretion is inhibited.

 4.   ADH acts on the distal renal tubules to increase their membrane permeability to water, thus increasing the rate of water reabsorption.

 5.   GI tract sensory receptors feed back the sensation of fullness to the hypothalamus, and under the influence of ADH, water is reabsorbed in the bowel.

   6.   The ICF volume in thirst center neurons increases, inhibiting the need to drink.

   7.   Together, the thirst feedback mechanisms and ADH function to conserve water and ensure its intake to maintain homeostasis.

 8.   The adrenals help control fluid and electrolyte balance through secretion of steroid hormones, mainly aldosterone.

Endocrine Organs and Their Function

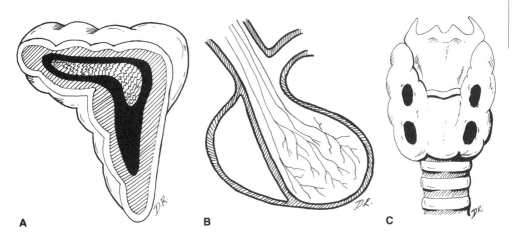

A　　　　　　　　　**B**　　　　　　　　　**C**

FIGURE 2-8.
(A) The adrenal glands. The adrenal glands help balance electrolytes by secreting steroid hormones. **(B) The pituitary gland.** The pituitary gland secretes antidiuretic hormone (ADH) that releases water in the kidney tubules. The pituitary also secretes adrenocorticotropin hormone (ACTH) that stimulates the adrenal glands. **(C) Parathyroid glands.** The parathyroid glands aid in maintaining electrolyte balance through secretion of parathyroid hormone (PTH).

　9. The parathyroid aids in maintaining electrolyte balance through secretion of parathyroid hormone, which regulates calcium balance.

10. Figure 2-8 provides more information on endocrine regulation.

D. Cardiovascular regulation

　1. The cardiovascular system regulates fluid volume, pressure sensors, and atrial natriuretic factor (Fig. 2-9).

2. Normal blood volume permits the heart to pump blood to the kidneys at an optimal pressure; adequate kidney perfusion allows urine to form.

3. Changes in blood volume directly affect arterial blood pressure and urinary output:

　　a. Increased blood volume increases cardiac output.

　　b. An increase in cardiac output causes arterial pressure to rise.

　　c. Elevations in arterial pressure directly affect the kidneys, causing an increase in urine output; a corresponding decrease in blood volume completes the feedback mechanism, thus maintaining a stable blood volume in spite of variations in daily intake.

4. Arterial baroreceptors and low-pressure sensors (stretch receptors) in the larger blood vessels (eg, aorta, carotids) respond to changes in blood volume:

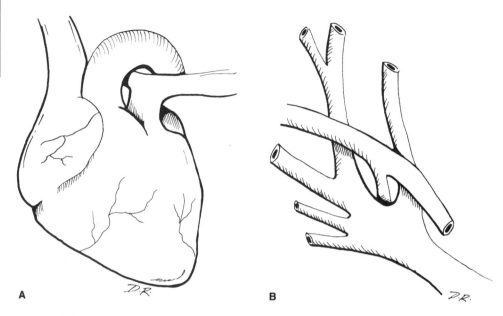

A   B

FIGURE 2-9.
(A) The heart. The heart regulates body fluids by propelling fluid through the body. **(B) The blood vessels.** Along with the heart, blood vessels help regulate fluid balance by vasoconstriction and vasodilation. Blood vessels contain pressure and stretch receptors that facilitate vasodilation and vasoconstriction.

    a.   A rise in arterial pressure causes the baroreceptors and stretch receptors to signal an inhibition of the sympathetic nervous system (SNS).

    b.   Reflex SNS inhibition causes dilation of renal arterioles with a subsequent increase in urine output.

    c.   Vasoconstriction or vasodilation will occur in response to arterial baroreceptor stimulation.

    5.   Atrial natriuretic factor (ANF) is a polypeptide hormone secreted by the cardiac atria into the blood following stretching of the atria by increased blood volume.

    6.   ANF signals the kidneys to decrease tubular reabsorption of sodium. As a result, urine osmolarity and output are significantly increased, reducing blood volume.

    7.   ANF has a short-term effect on blood volume; it appears to be counteracted by other regulatory mechanisms in chronic states of increased blood volume.

E.   **Gastrointestinal regulation**

    1.   The GI tract organs digest food (breaking it down chemically into simpler, soluble substances) so that it can be absorbed by body tissues.

     2.   **The hormonal and enzymatic processes involved in digestion, com-**

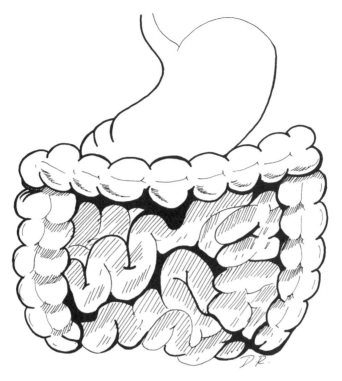

FIGURE 2-10.
Gastrointestinal organs. The stomach and intestines help balance the body's fluids and electrolytes by absorbing those that are needed and eliminating those that are not needed.

bined with passive and active transport, are the mechanisms through which the GI tract participates in fluid volume regulation (Fig. 2-10).

3. After initial gastric digestion, the fluid mixture of food, water, and GI tract secretions (a 24-hour volume of about 9 L) moves into the small intestine.

4. Approximately 85% to 95% of water absorption and most nutrient transport into the plasma volume takes place in the small intestine.

5. The colon absorbs additional water (500–1000 mL) and exchanges electrolytes before it moves the remaining waste matter toward the rectum and anus for eventual expulsion as feces.

F. Pulmonary regulation

1. The normal elimination of water through the lungs (insensible water loss) equals approximately 500 mL/d.

 2. **The amount of insensible water loss varies with hyperventilation and mechanical ventilation (Fig. 2-11).**

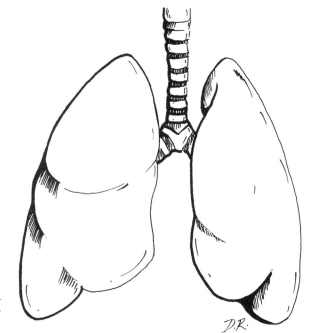

FIGURE 2-11.
The lungs. The lungs help balance body fluids since expired air is water saturated.

Bibliography

Bullock, B. (1996). *Pathophysiology: Adaptations and alterations in function* (4th ed.). Philadelphia: J. B. Lippincott.

Drummer, C., Gerzer, R., Heer, M. et al. (1992). Effects of an acute saline infusion on fluid and electrolyte metabolism in humans. *American Journal of Physiology,* May, 744–754.

Guyton, A. (1991). *Textbook of medical physiology* (8th ed.). Philadelphia: W. B. Saunders.

Kinney, M., Packa, D., & Dunbar, S. (1993). *AACN's clinical reference for critical-care nursing* (3rd ed.). St. Louis: C. V. Mosby.

Kokko, J., & Tannen, R. (1996). *Fluids and electrolytes* (3rd ed.). Philadelphia: W. B. Saunders.

Metheny, N. (1996). *Fluid and electrolyte balance: Nursing considerations* (3rd ed.) Philadelphia: J. B. Lippincott.

Miller, M. (1997). Fluid and electrolyte homeostasis in the elderly: Physiologic changes of aging and clinical consequences. *Baillieres Clinical Endocrinology and Metabolism,* 11(2), 367–387.

Narrins, R. (Ed). (1994). *Maxwell & Kleemans clinical disorders of fluid and electrolyte metabolism* (5th ed.). New York: McGraw-Hill.

Plante, G. E., Chakir, M., Lehoux, S., & Lortie, M. (1995). Disorders of body fluid balance: A new look into the mechanisms of disease. *Canadian Journal of Cardiology,* 11(9), 788–802.

Porth, C. (1994). *Pathophysiology: Concepts of altered health states* (4th ed.). Philadelphia: J. B. Lippincott.

Rose, B. (1994). *Clinical physiology of acid: base and electrolyte disorders* (4th ed.). New York: McGraw-Hill.

Seaman, S. L. (1995). *Renal physiology part II: Fluid and electrolyte regulation,* Neonatal Network, 14(5), 5–11.

Smith, K., & Brain, E. (1991). *Fluids and electrolytes: A conceptual approach* (2nd ed.). New York: Churchill Livingstone.

Szerlip, H., & Goldfarb, S. (1993). *Workshops in fluid and electrolyte disorders.* New York: Churchill Livingstone.

Toto, K. (1994). Endocrine physiology. *Critical Care Nursing Clinics of North America,* December, 647–657.

STUDY QUESTIONS

1. As part of the endocrine regulation of body fluid balance, osmoreceptor cells in the posterior hypothalamus secrete which of the following hormones when extracellular fluid (ECF) osmolarity increases?
   a. angiotensin I
   b. antidiuretic hormone (ADH)
   c. renin
   d. aldosterone

2. Which of the following body systems is *not* a primary systemic regulator of body fluids?
   a. renal system
   b. gastrointestinal system
   c. respiratory system
   d. cardiovascular system

3. Capillary dynamics are directly related to the hydrostatic pressure differences between:
   a. intracellular fluid (ICF) and extracellular fluid (ECF)
   b. venous and arterial ends of capillaries
   c. osmosis and diffusion
   d. filtration and capillaries

4. The mechanism by which glucose and most amino acids are able to diffuse into and out of cells is termed:
   a. hydrostatic pressure
   b. Starling's law
   c. facilitated diffusion
   d. colloidal osmotic pressure

5. The difference between active and passive transport involves:
   a. the type of solute
   b. pressure gradients
   c. thickness of the capillary wall
   d. expenditure of cellular energy

6. Which of the following disease states can cause excessive insensible fluid loss?
   a. vomiting
   b. diuretic therapy
   c. diarrhea
   d. fever with diaphoresis

7. The pumping action of the heart generates:
   a. hydrostatic pressure
   b. osmotic pressure
   c. oncotic pressure
   d. hypertonic pressure

8. The sodium-potassium pump plays a key role in maintaining the volume of:
   a. ECF
   b. ICF
   c. intravascular fluid
   d. interstitial fluid

9. When performing a complete fluid and electrolyte assessment, the nurse should evaluate a patient's protein levels because proteins are responsible for:
   a. anticoagulation effects
   b. vascular and cell wall integrity
   c. fluid movement outside of the cell
   d. immunosuppressive defenses

10. Which of the following hormones does *not* help balance the body's fluids?
    a. renin
    b. aldosterone
    c. parathyroid hormone (PTH)
    d. antidiuretic hormone (ADH)

11. Hormonal and enzymatic processes, active and passive transport describe mechanisms of fluid/electrolyte balance in which organ system:
    a. renal
    b. endocrine
    c. gastrointestinal
    d. respiratory

12. A disorder of which organ can result in changes in serum calcium levels:
    a. heart
    b. lungs
    c. kidney
    d. parathyroid

ANSWER KEY

Question	Correct answer	Correct answer rationale	Incorrect answer rationales
1.	b	ADH is secreted by the pituitary when signaled by the hypothalamus that ECF osmolarity has increased. As a result, increased water will be reabsorbed in the kidneys, thus decreasing ECF osmolarity.	a, c, and d. Angiotensin I, renin, and aldosterone are part of the renal regulation of fluid balance.
2.	b	The respiratory system is not a primary systemic regulator of fluid balance.	a, c, and d. The renal, gastrointestinal, and cardiovascular systems, as well as endocrine system, are the primary systemic body fluid regulators.
3.	b	Capillary dynamics are directly related to the hydrostatic pressure differences between the venous and arterial ends of capillaries and aid in fluid exchange between the intravascular and interstitial spaces.	a, c, and d. These responses are incorrect because they do not reflect the differences in capillary dynamics.
4.	c	Facilitated diffusion is a specialized type of passive transport requiring the participation of a carrier protein for some substances to cross semipermeable membranes. It is the mechanism by which glucose and most amino acids are able to diffuse into and out of cells.	a, b, and d. These responses are incorrect because they do not reflect the movement of molecules into and out of the cells.
5.	d	Active transport differs from passive transport in that cellular energy is required to fuel these pumps and permit substances to move against pressure gradients.	a, b, and c. These responses are incorrect.
6.	d	Fever with diaphoresis will cause excessive fluid loss through the skin. Since this loss is not measurable, it is an insensible fluid loss.	a, b, and c. These states will cause abnormal and excessive fluid loss, but these losses are measurable and therefore are not insensible.
7.	a	The pumping action of the heart is hydrostatic pressure (pressure of a fluid mass pushing outward against the boundaries of its container).	b. Osmotic pressure refers to the pressure inside the ECF and ICF. c. This response is incorrect. d. There is no such entity as hypertonic pressure.
8.	b	The sodium-potassium pump plays a key role in the maintenance of ICF volume. The outflow of sodium ions counter balances the osmotic pressure exerted by the intracellular proteins to pull excess water into the cells.	a, c, and d. These represent the other fluid compartments in which the sodium-potassium pump has a lesser influence.

Question	Correct answer	Correct answer rationale	Incorrect answer rationales
9.	b	Plasma proteins, particularly albumin, maintain cell wall integrity and blood vessel integrity, keeping fluid inside the fluid compartments.	a. The plasma protein fibrinogen is responsible for blood clotting. c. Proteins prevent fluid from moving outside of the cell. d. The plasma protein globulin is responsible for keeping the immune system intact.
10.	c	Parathyroid hormone (PTH) does not play a role in fluid balance.	a and b. The renin-angiotensin-aldosterone mechanism plays a critical role in fluid balance. d. Antidiuretic hormone (ADH) helps regulate fluid balance by reabsorbing water in the renal tubules.
11.	c	The gastrointestinal system helps in the balance of fluids and electrolytes through these mechanisms.	a, b, and d. These organs help balance fluids and electrolytes through mechanisms not described here.
12.	d	The parathyroid glands are responsible for the balance of serum calcium.	a, b, and c. These organs are not responsible for calcium balance.

3

Alterations in
Fluid Balance

I. **Alterations in body fluid balance**

A. Fluid volume deficit (FVD)

1. FVD, commonly called *hypovolemia* or dehydration, is a condition in which fluid loss exceeds fluid intake.
2. FVD may be isotonic, hypotonic, or hypertonic.

31

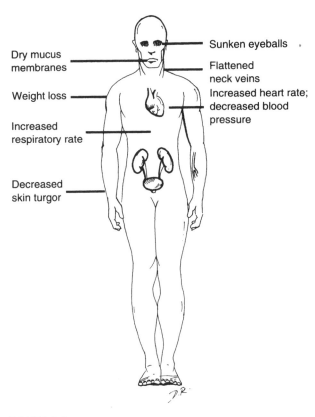

Dry mucus membranes

Sunken eyeballs

Flattened neck veins

Weight loss

Increased heart rate; decreased blood pressure

Increased respiratory rate

Decreased skin turgor

FIGURE 3-1.
Fluid volume deficit.

3. Figure 3-1 illustrates some symptoms of FVD.

B. Fluid volume excess (FVE)

1. **FVE, commonly called *hypervolemia*, is a condition in which fluid intake exceeds fluid loss.**

2. **FVE is dangerous because it can lead to congestive heart failure.**

3. FVE may be isotonic, hypotonic, or hypertonic.

4. Figure 3-2 illustrates some symptoms of FVE.

II.   Isotonic FVD

A. Description

1. Isotonic FVD is an equal decrease in Extracellular Fluid (ECF) solute concentration (especially sodium) and water volume. This means that fluids, electrolytes, and other solutes are lost in equal amounts.

2. The ECF maintains its normal iso-osmolar state.

3. No changes are produced in the ICF volume.

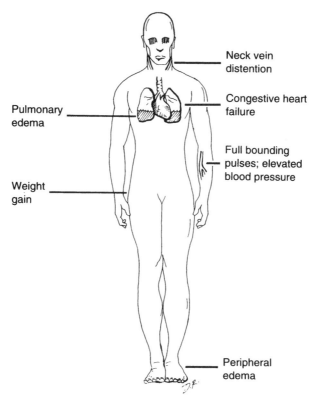

FIGURE 3-2.
Fluid volume excess.

B. Etiology

1. Isotonic FVD *can* result from excessive loss of iso-osmolar fluids through:
   a. GI tract (through vomiting, diarrhea, nasogastric suctioning)
   b. Kidneys (through diuresis secondary to renal disease and diuretic use)
   c. Skin (through excessive perspiration and burns)
   d. Hemorrhage

2. Lack of intake of fluids and electrolytes may occur secondary to an inability to ingest orally (eg, decreased level of consciousness, sedation, nothing-by-mouth status).

3. Iso-osmolar fluid shifts into potential anatomic body spaces (eg, peritoneal cavity, interstitial fluid compartment) where the fluid is not readily available for exchange with the plasma volume. The interstitial space is the most common site for third spacing.

4. **This phenomenon of fluid shifting into spaces other than the ECF or ICF is known as *third spacing* and is seen as edema. The danger of third spacing is that the fluid leaves the circulatory system and is un-**

available for the transport of oxygen and nutrients. **In third spacing, the patient can be edematous but the intravascular space can be dehydrated.** It can occur secondary to:
   a.   Acute bowel obstruction
   b.   Infection that leads to sepsis (eg, peritonitis)
   c.   Blockage of the lymphatic drainage system
   d.   Liver disease (eg, cirrhosis)
   e.   Poor circulation

C.   **Assessment findings**
   1.   Clinical manifestations of isotonic FVD may include:
      a.   Acute weight loss (especially if greater than 5% of total body weight)
      b.   Cardiovascular changes (eg, increased heart rate, decreased blood pressure [especially if resulting in postural hypotension], and flattened neck veins in the supine position)
      c.   Increased respiratory rate
      d.   Decreased hydration of the skin and mucous membranes (eg, dry tongue, "sticky" mucous membranes in the oral cavity, and decreased skin turgor)
      e.   Decreased and concentrated urine output
      f.   Increased hematocrit
      g.   Thick and sticky respiratory secretions
      h.   Sunken eyeballs

   2.   **Symptoms and consequences of third-space fluid accumulation depend on the location of the space:**
      a.   **Ascites is fluid accumulation in the peritoneal cavity; it is marked by increased abdominal girth.**
      b.   **Pleural effusion is fluid in the pleural space. Auscultation of the lungs in the area of the effusion reveals decreased breath sounds; the patient also may experience shortness of breath.**
      c.   **Pericardial effusion results from fluid accumulation in the pericardial cavity; it is manifested by altered hemodynamics and muffled heart sounds. This can be life threatening as the fluid can crush the heart.**
      d.   **Edema in the feet (pedal) that works its way up the extremities is the most common. This can cause significant discomfort to the patient.**
      e.   **Anasarca is generalized third spacing that affects the whole body.**
      f.   **Pulmonary edema, which is life threatening, is fluid accumulation in the interstitial spaces in the lung.**
   3.   In third-space fluid accumulation, weight *gain* may occur in spite of the fluid deficit in the intravascular space.

D.   **Potential nursing diagnoses**
   1.   Fluid Volume Deficit
   2.   Altered Tissue Perfusion (the kidneys are at special risk)
   3.   High Risk for Injury
   4.   Ineffective Breathing Patterns
   5.   Decreased Cardiac Output

6. Altered Nutrition: Less Than Body Requirements
7. Altered Oral Mucous Membranes
8. Risk for Impaired Skin Integrity
9. Fatigue
10. Risk for Activity Intolerance

E. **Interventions**

1. Medical management involves:
   a. Replacement with isotonic fluids and electrolytes by oral or IV route
   b. IV replacement of blood, blood components, or proteins if the FVD is due to hemorrhage or fluid shift to the tissues
   c. Treatment of contributory underlying disease states (eg, prescription of medications to counteract vomiting or diarrhea)
   d. Removal of third space fluid accumulations by direct drainage (eg, chest tube insertion to drain a pleural effusion) when indicated
   e. Mobilization of interstitial fluids (must be done with great caution because this can lead to FVE)

2. Nursing considerations
   a. Assess cardiovascular, respiratory, and neurologic status.
   b. Assess skin turgor and hydration of mucous membranes.
   c. Monitor laboratory values (eg, hematocrit, hemoglobin, blood urea nitrogen [BUN]).
   d. Monitor intake and output; urine output should be a bare minimum of approximately 30 mL/h or about 500 to 700 mL/d.
   e. Monitor weight daily; weight loss of more than 0.5 lb/d is considered fluid loss.
   f. Provide patient teaching about medication regimen, prescribed diet and foods to avoid, signs and symptoms of the specific disorder for which the patient is at risk (eg, weight loss), and preventive measures.

F. **Evaluation**

1. The patient's pulse, blood pressure, and neck veins are normal.
2. The patient's tongue and mucous membranes are moist, and skin turgor is good.
3. The patient's hematocrit is increased.
4. The patient's breath sounds are clear.
5. Perfusion of vital organs is maintained.
6. The patient is free from injury.
7. The quantity and characteristics of urinary output are normal.

III. Hypotonic FVD

A. **Description**

1. **Hypotonic FVD is a decrease in solute concentration with water volume remaining normal. This means that electrolytes and other solutes are lost in excess of water.**
2. The ECF is hypo-osmolar, and fluid shifts into the cells.

B. Etiology

1. GI fluid loss through vomiting and diarrhea
2. Renal loss
3. Malnutrition
4. Iatrogenic fluid replacement with hypotonic fluid solutions

C. Assessment findings

1. Symptoms of hypotonic FVD are the same as for isotonic FVD (see Section II.C).
2. Additional symptoms can include:
    a. Weakness
    b. Fatigue
    c. Muscle cramps
    d. Postural hypotension
    e. Confusion

D. Potential nursing diagnoses (same as for isotonic FVD, see Section II.D)

E. Interventions

1. **Medical management involves the same treatments as for isotonic FVD (see Section II.E.1), except for fluid replacement strategies:**
    a. **For mild hyponatremia, replacement with oral salt and water or IV isotonic saline**
    b. **For severe hyponatremia, replacement with hypertonic saline solutions**
    c. **Replacement of potassium, if depleted.**
2. Nursing considerations are the same as for isotonic FVD (see Section II.E.2).

F. Evaluation

1. Serum sodium level returns to normal.
2. The evaluation is the same as for isotonic FVD (see Section II.F.).

IV. Hypertonic FVD

A. Description

1. Hypertonic FVD is a decrease in water volume without a corresponding decrease in solute concentration. This means that water is lost in excess of electrolytes and other solutes.
2. The ECF is hyperosmolar.
3. ICF shifts into the extracellular compartment.

B. Etiology

1. Osmotic diuresis or severe GI infections causing ECF volume depletion and increased sodium concentration
2. Poorly regulated nasogastric tube feedings
3. Insensible water loss during prolonged fever
4. Altered mental status in which a person is unable to access water freely; a person with an intact sensorium, normal thirst regulation, and uninhibited water access cannot usually develop a hypertonic FVD.
5. Impaired thirst regulation, possibly due to a hypothalamic lesion

C. **Assessment findings**
1. Decreased skin turgor
2. Decreased hydration of mucous membranes
3. Decreased blood pressure, increased pulse, postural hypotension
4. Increased thirst
5. Pitting edema
6. Increased respiratory rate and depth
7. Decreased peripheral pulses
8. Hyperactive deep tendon reflexes

D. **Potential nursing diagnoses (same as for isotonic FVD, see Section II.D)**

E. **Interventions**

1. **Medical management involves treating the underlying disease process and replacing fluid loss:**
   a. **For water loss, replace with water only**
   b. **For sodium loss, replace with dilute (hypotonic) saline IV**
2. Nursing considerations are the same as for isotonic FVD (see Section II.E.2).

F. **Evaluation**
1. The patient's vital signs, skin turgor, and mucous membranes are normal.
2. The patient breathes normally.
3. The patient displays no signs of edema.
4. Vital signs are normal.

V. Isotonic FVE

A. **Description**

1. **Isotonic FVE is an increase in water volume and solute concentration (especially sodium) in the ECF in proportions equal to its normal iso-osmolar state.**
2. It does not involve an ICF shift.

B. **Etiology**
1. Excessive intake of sodium and water, either orally or IV
2. Iso-osmolar fluid retention secondary to impaired regulatory mechanisms (eg, renal dysfunction, inappropriate secretion of ADH, cardiac disease)
3. Use of corticosteroids
4. Chronic liver failure

C. **Assessment findings**
1. Clinical manifestations include:
   a. Circulatory overload
   b. Interstitial edema
   c. Rapid weight gain (especially if greater than 5% of total body weight)
2. In patients with circulatory overload:
   a. Increased plasma volume increases mean arterial pressure. The myocardium stretches to accommodate the larger blood volume, the

cardiac output is correspondingly increased, and plasma hydrostatic pressure also increases beyond normal values.

b. If cardiac status is compromised or if the isotonic hypervolemia continues for a prolonged period, the heart cannot handle the excess volume. This results in congestive heart failure (CHF) and edema.

c. When a patient's intravascular space becomes overloaded with fluid, eventually the heart will not be able to accommodate the blood.

d. As a result of CHF, the FVE progresses into the pulmonary edema, which is life-threatening.

e. Symptoms include elevated blood pressure, bounding pulse, and neck vein distention.

2. In patients with interstitial edema:

a. A higher plasma hydrostatic pressure forces a higher-than-normal outflow of fluid from the capillaries into the tissue spaces.

b. Fluid can accumulate subcutaneously in dependent parts of the body; this is peripheral edema.

c. Fluid accumulating in the lungs is heard as moist crackles on auscultation.

D.   Potential nursing diagnoses

1. Fluid Volume Excess
2. High Risk for Ineffective Breathing Pattern
3. Decreased Cardiac Output
4. Impaired Gas Exchange
5. Risk for Suffocation
6. Ineffective Breathing Pattern
7. Ineffective Airway Clearance
8. Inability to Sustain Spontaneous Ventilation
9. Dysfunctional Ventilatory Weaning Response
10. Anxiety

E.   Interventions

1. Medical management involves:

a. Prescription of diuretics to enhance water excretion by the kidneys

b. Restriction of oral fluid and salt intake

c. Titration of IV fluid volume composition and intake

d. Treatment of contributory underlying disease states (eg, in CHF, digoxin would be prescribed to increase cardiac output)

2. Nursing considerations:

a. Assess cardiovascular status (eg, pulse rate and quality, blood pressure, neck vein filling).

b. Monitor hemodynamic parameters, such as cardiac output and intracardiac pressures.

c. Assess respiratory status; auscultate breath sounds, and monitor rate and ease of breathing.

d. Monitor for weight gain in relation to total body weight; estimate a gain of 1 L of fluid for every kilogram (2.2 lb) of increased weight.

e. Measure and record daily weights.

f. Monitor for the presence of peripheral edema. Check for pitting edema by pressing gently with a fingertip into edematous area; if depression remains, the depth of the "pit" indicates severity of the edema.

g. Monitor laboratory values; decreased hematocrit and BUN may indicate isotonic FVE.

h. Monitor intake and output.

i. Position the patient comfortably to relieve respiratory symptoms, edema, and pressure.

j. Evaluate the patient's knowledge of the prescribed diet or medication regimen; assess for any dietary factors that may have led to FVE.

k. Refer the patient to a dietitian for nutritional consultation.

F. Evaluation

1. The patient's breath sounds, breathing patterns, vital signs, and urinary output are normal.

2. The patient displays no signs of edema.

3. The patient's fluid volume status is normal.

4. The patient's cardiac output is normal.

VI. Hypotonic FVE

A. Description

1. **Hypotonic FVE, sometimes called *water intoxication*, is an increase in water volume without a corresponding increase in sodium concentration, producing hypo-osmolar ECF.**

2. Fluid shifts into the cells from the ECF, causing waterlogging of cells.

B. Etiology

1. Hypotonic FVE results from:

a. Excess oral intake of water or IV fluid therapy with hypotonic solutions (eg, 5% dextrose and water)

b. Underlying medical conditions that impair normal fluid excretion, including cardiac disease (in which there is insufficient arterial pressure for normal renal perfusion); syndrome of inappropriate ADH (SIADH) secretion resulting from extreme stress, benign and cancerous central nervous system (CNS) lesions, or fever; overuse of drugs, such as cortico-steroids

c. Loss of isotonic fluids (through vomiting, burns, hemorrhage) combined with replacement of water but not sodium and other lost solutes

2. Hypotonic FVE always involves an osmotic fluid shift from the ECF into the ICF (cell swelling).

C. Assessment findings

1. Weight gain

2. Thirst

3. Excretion of dilute urine

4. Nonpitting edema

5. Dysrythmias secondary to decreased plasma sodium and potassium

6. Low sodium levels

7.   Symptoms of cerebral ICF excess occurrs as water shifts into the cells of the brain, including:
a.   Nausea
b.   Malaise
c.   Lethargy
d.   Headache
e.   Seizures, coma, and death if ICF fluid shift into brain cells is not reversed.

D.   Potential nursing diagnoses
1.   Fluid Volume Excess
2.   High Risk for Ineffective Breathing Pattern
3.   Decreased Cardiac Output
4.   Impaired Gas Exchange
5.   Risk for Suffocation
6.   Ineffective Breathing Pattern
7.   Ineffective Airway Clearance
8.   Inability to Sustain Spontaneous Ventilation
9.   Dysfunctional Ventilatory Weaning Response
10.   Anxiety

E.   Interventions
1.   Medical management involves:
a.   Restricting water intake to a volume that is less than urine output
b.   Increasing salt in the diet
c.   Administering IV hypertonic (3%) saline solutions for severe hyponatremia (eg, sodium concentration of 110 mEq/L or less). Note that hypertonic solutions are only given if the patient's life is threatened and should be used cautiously to avoid overcorrection of the sodium loss; plasma sodium should not rise above 145 to 150 mEq/L.
2.   Nursing considerations are the same as for isotonic FVE (see Section V.E.2), plus the following:
a.   Monitor for abnormal water-seeking behavior such as may be seen in patients with psychological disorders (psychogenic polydipsia) or in those whose thirst regulation has been altered by disease process (primary polydipsia).
b.   Assess neurologic status for signs of ICF excess.

F.   Evaluation
1.   The patient's urinary output and cardiac output are normal.
2.   The patient's level of consciousness is normal.
3.   The patient is free from injury.
4.   Sodium levels are normal.

VII.   Hypertonic FVE

A.   Description
1.   Hypertonic FVE is an increase in sodium concentration with water volume remaining normal.

2. This results in ECF that is hyperosmolar compared with normal plasma and tissue fluids.
3. ICF shifts into the ECF.

B. Etiology
  1. Hypertonic FVE results from:
     a. Excess intake of hypertonic fluids, such as salty liquids or seawater
     b. Excess solute (eg, sodium) retention secondary to impaired regulatory mechanisms or disease process.
  2. It always involves an osmotic fluid shift from the ICF to the ECF (cell shrinkage).

C. Assessment findings
  1. Clinical manifestations relate to the effect of the excess solute in the ECF combined with FVE; symptoms of hypertonic FVE are the same as for isotonic FVE (see Section V.C).
  2. ICF deficit is manifested by neurologic symptoms (eg, decreased level of consciousness [LOC], lethargy, muscle twitching, possible seizures, and coma); symptom severity is related to the speed with which plasma sodium concentration rises, with its subsequent osmotic dehydration of cerebral cells.
  3. Hypernatremia is present.

D. Potential nursing diagnoses
  1. Fluid Volume Excess
  2. High Risk for Ineffective Breathing Pattern
  3. Decreased Cardiac Output
  4. Impaired Gas Exchange
  5. Risk for Suffocation
  6. Ineffective Breathing Pattern
  7. Ineffective Airway Clearance
  8. Inability to Sustain Spontaneous Ventilation
  9. Dysfunctional Ventilatory Weaning Response
  10. Anxiety

E. Interventions
  1. Medical management involves:
     a. Treating underlying disease (eg, renal failure or CNS lesion)
     b. Discontinuing or removing the source of the hypertonic fluid intake
     c. Removing excess sodium by diuretics
     d. Correcting the ICF water deficit (plus water lost with diuretic therapy) through replacement with oral water or hypotonic IV solution
     e. Treatment of the symptoms of the high ECF solute and the ICF deficit
  2. Nursing considerations are the same as for isotonic FVE (see Section V.E.2), plus the following:
     a. Assess LOC, neuromuscular status, presence or absence of tremors, and rigidity to detect any signs of ICF deficit.
     b. Provide patient teaching regarding prevention through dietary modifications, avoidance of high-salt foods, and self-monitoring of symptoms (eg, rapid weight gain, presence of edema).

TABLE 3-1

Changes in extracellular fluid volume and plasma sodium concentration as determinants of body fluid balance

TYPE OF ECF FLUID VOLUME IMBALANCE	ECF VOLUME	ECF SOLUTE CONCENTRATION Na+ (mEq)	ICF VOLUME (CELLS SWELL OR SHRINK)	ICF SOLUTE CONCENTRATION K+ (mEq)
Isotonic FVE H₂O gain = Na+ gain	↑	No change	No change	No change
Hypertonic FVE Na+ gain > H₂O gain	↑	↑	*Cells shrink*	↑
Hypertonic FVE H₂O gain > Na+ gain	↑	↓	*Cells swell*	↓
Isotonic FVD H₂O loss = Na+ loss	↓	No change	No change	No change
Hypertonic FVD H₂O loss > Na+ loss	↓	↑	*Cells shrink*	↑
Hypotonic FVD Na+ loss > H2O loss	↓	↓	*Cells swell*	↓

Key: ECF, extracellular fluid; ICF, intracellular fluid; FVE, fluid volume excess; FVD, fluid volume deficit.

F. Evaluation

1. The patient's LOC is normal.
2. The patient's urinary output, vital signs, and breath sounds are normal.
3. The patient's fluid volume status is normal.
4. The patient's cardiac output is normal.
5. The patient is free from injury. (Table 3.1 illustrates changes in extracellular volume and concentrations.)

Bibliography

Bullock, B. (1996). *Pathophysiology: Adaptations and alterations in function* (4th ed.). Philadelphia: J. B. Lippincott.

Drummer, C., Gerzer, R., Heer, M., et al. (1992). Effects of an acute saline infusion on fluid and electrolyte metabolism in humans. *American Journal of Physiology,* May, 744–754.

Guyton, A. (1991). *Textbook of medical physiology.* (8th ed.). Philadelphia: W. B. Saunders.

Kinney, M., Packa, D., & Dunbar, S. (1993). *AACN's clinical reference for critical-care nursing* (3rd ed.). St. Louis: C.V. Mosby.

Kokko, J., & Tannen, R. (1996). *Fluids and electrolytes* (3rd ed.). Philadelphia: W. B. Saunders.

Metheny, N. (1996). *Fluid and electrolyte balance: Nursing considerations* (3rd ed.). Philadelphia: J. B. Lippincott.

Miller, M. (1997). Fluid and electrolyte homeostasis in the elderly: physiologic changes of aging and clinical consequences. *Baillieres Clinical Endocrinology and Metabolism,* 11(2), 367–387.

Narrins, R. (Ed). (1994). *Maxwell & Kleemans clinical disorders of fluid and electrolyte metabolism* (5th ed.). New York: McGraw-Hill.

North American Nursing Diagnosis Association. Nursing Diagnosis: Definitions and Classifications. The Auth. 1996.

Plante, G. E., Chakir, M., Lehoux, S., & Lortie, M. (1995). Disorders of body fluid balance: A new look into the mechanisms of disease. *Canadian Journal of Cardiology,* 11(9), 788–802.

Porth, C. (1994). *Pathophysiology: Concepts of altered health states* (4th ed.). Philadelphia: J. B. Lippincott.

Rose, B. (1994). *Clinical physiology of acid-base and electrolyte disorders* (4th ed.). New York: McGraw-Hill.

Seaman, S. L. (1995). Renal physiology part II: Fluid and electrolyte regulation. *Neonatal network,* 14(5), 5–11.

Smith, K., & Brain, E. (1991). *Fluids and electrolytes: A conceptual approach* (2nd ed.). New York: Churchill Livingstone.

Szerlip, H., & Goldfarb, S. (1993). *Workshops in fluid and electrolyte disorders.* New York: Churchill Livingstone.

Toto, K. (1994). Endocrine physiology. *Critical Care Nursing Clinics of North America,* December, 647–657.

STUDY QUESTIONS

1. In which of the following types of fluid volume deficit (FVD) does water volume remain normal?
   a. isotonic FVD
   b. hypotonic FVD
   c. hypertonic FVD
   d. allatonic FVD

2. When monitoring a patient with a isotonic FVD, the nurse is aware that the minimum urine output is:
   a. 10 mL/hour
   b. 20 mL/hour
   c. 30 mL/hour
   d. 40 mL/hour

3. The phenomenon of third-space fluid shifting involves:
   a. iso-osmolar fluid shifts into body cavities where the fluid is not available for exchange with plasma volume
   b. the three types of fluid volume deficits
   c. hypo-osmolar fluid shifts into the extracellular fluid
   d. iatrogenic fluid shifts into the lymphatic system

4. In patients with isotonic fluid volume excess (FVE) and circulating overload, the potential outcome is:
   a. cell swelling
   b. cerebral cell dehydration
   c. water intoxication
   d. congestive heart failure (CHF)

5. The physician has ordered administration of a hypertonic saline solution. The nurse would administer:
   a. 3% saline solution
   b. 0.33% saline solution
   c. 0.45% saline solution
   d. 0.9% saline solution

6. Third-space fluid accumulation may occur in the:
   a. peritoneal cavity
   b. pleural space
   c. interstitial space
   d. all of the above

7. Which of the following is a potential nursing diagnosis for a patient with isotonic FVD?
   a. increased cardiac output
   b. decreased cardiac output
   c. fluid volume excess
   d. altered urinary habits

8. When assessing a patient with hypotonic FVE, the nurse can expect to find:
   a. hyponatremia
   b. confusion
   c. headache
   d. all of the above

9. In evaluating nursing intervention for hypotonic fluid volume excess, the nurse knows that her interventions are effective if which of the following is present:
   a. hyponatremia
   b. dilute urine
   c. nonpitting edema
   d. normal level of consciousness

10. Which is the most important parameter to evaluate when assessing a patients hydration status:
    a. respirations
    b. mobility
    c. quality and character of urine
    d. pulse

ANSWER KEY

Question	Correct answer	Correct answer rationale	Incorrect answer rationales
1.	b	Hypotonic FVD involves a decrease in solute concentration with water volume remaining normal.	a. Isotonic FVD involves an equal decrease in ECF solute concentration and water volume. c. Hypertonic FVD involves a decrease in water volume without a corresponding decrease in solute concentration. d. There is no such entity.
2.	c	Urine output should be a bare minimum of 30 ml/hour or 500 to 700 ml/day.	a, b, and d. These responses are incorrect because the proper amount is described above.
3.	a	Third-space fluid shifting involves iso-osmolar fluid shifts into spaces other than the ICF or ECF where the fluid is not available for exchanges with plasma.	b, c, and d. These responses do not reflect third spacing.
4.	d	In patients with circulatory overload due to isotonic FVE, the excess volume cannot be managed and results in CHF and edema.	a. Cell shrinking, not swelling, occurs. b and c. These responses are incorrect.
5.	a	Hypertonic fluid has a greater concentration of sodium to water volume.	b, c, and d. A 3% saline solution has has a higher concentration than a 0.33%, 0.45%, or 0.9% saline solution.
6.	d	Third-space fluid accumulation refers to the accumulation of fluid in spaces that are not part of the circulation. These spaces include the peritoneal cavity, pleural space, and interstitial space.	
7.	b	Isotonic FVD may change cardiac output because as fluid is lost, cardiac output tends to drop. Assessment findings characteristic of FVD could also include decreased blood pressure and tachycardia.	a. This response is incorrect. c. Fluid volume excess is the direct opposite of fluid volume deficit. d. Altered urinary habits is not a potential nursing diagnosis.
8.	d	Symptoms of hypotonic FVE are hyponatremia, confusion, and headache. Other symptoms include nausea, malaise, lethargy, weight gain, thirst, and nonpitting edema.	See correct answer.

Question	Correct answer	Correct answer rationale	Incorrect answer rationales
9.	d	A normal level of consciousness indicates that the therapy is effective. Hypotonic FVE causes "water-logging" of cerebral brain cells.	a, b, and c. These are signs of FVE.
10.	c	When hydration is normal, the urine output will be at least 30 cc's per hour and the color normal.	a, b, and c. These parameters are always important to assess, but letter c is the best answer because it more appropriately reflects hydration.

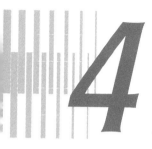

Electrolyte Balance

I. Overview of electrolytes

A. Description
1. Electrolytes are solutes that are found in body fluids (eg, intracellular fluid [ICF] and extracellular fluid [ECF]).

 2. Electrolytes develop an electrical charge when dissolved in water:
   a. Positively charged ions are called *cations.*
   b. Negatively charged ions are called *anions.*
3. Major body electrolytes include:
   a. Sodium (Na^+)—cation
   b. Potassium (K^+)—cation
   c. Chloride (Cl^-)—anion
   d. Calcium (Ca^+)—cation
   e. Magnesium (Mg^+)—cation
   f. Phosphorus (P^-)—anion
   g. Hydrogen (H^+)—cation
   h. Bicarbonate (HCO_3^-)—anion

B. Sources of electrolytes
1. Normal sources of electrolyte intake include all foods and fluids.
2. Abnormal sources of electrolyte intake include:
   a. Medications

b.   Intravenous solutions

c.   Hyperalimentation

C.   Role of electrolytes

1.   Electrolytes conduct electricity across cell membranes; they are needed for life processes to occur.

2.   Electrolytes function to:

a.   Maintain osmolality of body fluid compartments

b.   Regulate balance of acids and bases

c.   Aid in neurologic and neuromuscular conduction

D.   Balance of electrolytes

1.   **For a homeostatic condition to exist, equal amounts of anions and cations must be present on either side of the cell membrane (Fig. 4-1); this is known as electrical neutrality.**

2.   Electrolytes will move from one side of the cell membrane to another in an attempt to maintain an electrically neutral state.

3.   Extracellular electrolytes are found in the interstitial and intravascular fluids where there is a balance of cations and anions.

4.   Intracellular electrolytes are found in the intercellular space where there is a balance of cations and anions.

II.   Electrolyte distribution and excretion

A.   Distribution

1.   Electrolyte distribution varies between the ICF and ECF

2.   ICF electrolytes include:

a.   Potassium, the chief cation

b.   Phosphorus, the chief anion

c.   Large amount of protein

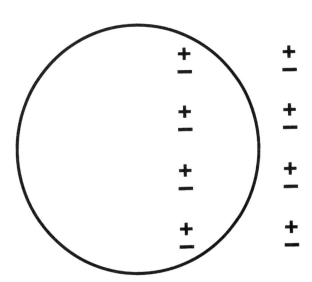

FIGURE 4-1.
Electrical neutrality.

       d.   Small amounts of magnesium, calcium, sulfate, and bicarbonate (See Table 1-2).

       e.   Extremely small amounts of sodium and chloride

   3. ECF electrolytes include:

       a.   Sodium, the chief cation

       b.   Chloride, the chief anion

       c.   Bicarbonate

       d.   Small amounts of potassium, calcium, magnesium, sulfate, and phosphorus

       e.   Protein in an amount smaller than in the ECF (Table 1-1).

   5. The concentration of electrolytes in body fluids can be expressed as *milliequivalents per liter* (mEq/L) or *milligrams per deciliter* (mg/dL).

   6. The ECF includes intravascular and interstitial fluids; the interstitial fluid has essentially the same electrolyte distribution as the intravascular fluid, but it is not measurable.

   7. ICF electrolytes are found in the intracellular space only and are not measurable; their values can be inferred only from ECF values.

   8. The concentration of specific electrolytes can be measured using serum or urine tests (Table 4-1).

B.   **Excretion**

   1. Electrolytes are lost during excessive elimination of body fluids for any reason.

   2. Renal excretion of electrolytes is abnormal when diuretics are used.

   3. Gastrointestinal (GI) elimination of electrolytes is abnormal when diarrhea is present.

   4. **In upper GI tract fluid elimination, hydrogen and potassium tend to be lost.**

   5. In lower GI tract fluid elimination, bicarbonate tends to be lost.

   6. Excessive diaphoresis contributes to sodium and chloride loss.

   7. Surgical drains also may contribute to excessive electrolyte loss.

III. Electrolyte regulation

A.   **Renal regulation**

   1. Electrolytes are regulated mainly by the kidneys and the endocrine system.

   2. **In the kidneys, electrolytes are balanced by glomerular filtration, tubular reabsorption, and secretion.**

       a.   The process of glomerular filtration can be compared to filtration that occurs outside of the body (ie, filtration of coffee).

       b.   Water goes through the filter and takes smaller substances along with it, leaving the larger substances behind in the filter (ie, in the example of coffee filter, water will take the color and flavor of the coffee, leaving the larger grounds behind in the filter).

       c.   The glomerulus provides the same functions.

       d.   It is a filter that leaves the larger molecules (protein, red and white blood cells) in the bloodstream while filtering out the smaller molecules (electrolytes, waste products).

TABLE 4-1

Laboratory Tests Used to Evaluate Fluid and Electrolyte Status

TEST	USUAL REFERENCE RANGE	SI UNITS
Serum sodium	135–145 mEq/L	135–145 mmol/L
Serum potassium	3.5–5.5 mEq/L	3.5–5.5 mmol/L
Total serum calcium	8.5–10.5 mg/dl (approximately 50% in ionized form)	2.1–2.6 mmol/L
Serum magnesium	1.5–2.5 mEq/L	0.80–1.2 mmol/L
Serum phosphorus	2.5–4.5 mEq/L	0.80–1.5 mmol/L
Serum chloride	100–106 mEq/L	100–106 mmol/L
Carbon dioxide content	24–30 mEq/L	24–30 mmol/L
Serum osmolality	280–295 mOsm/kg	280–295 mmol/L
Blood urea nitrogen (BUN)	10–20 mg/dl	3.5–7 mmol/L of urea
Serum creatinine	0.7–1.5 mg/dl	60–130 umol/L
BUN to creatinine ratio	10:1	
Hematocrit	Male: 44–52%	Volume fraction: 0.44–0.52
	Female: 39–47%	Volume fraction: 0.39–0.47
Serum glucose	70–110 mg/dl	3.9–6.1 mmol/L
Serum albumin	3.5–5.5 g/dl	3.5–5.5 g/L
Urinary sodium	80–180 mEq/day	80–180 mmol/day
Urinary potassium	40–80 mEq/day	40–80 mmol/day
Urinary chloride	110–250 mEq/day	110–250 mmol/day
Urinary specific gravity	1.025–1.035 = physiologic range after fluid restriction	1.025–1.035
	1.010–1.020 = random specimen with normal fluid intake	
Urine osmolality		
Extrreme range	50–1400 mOsm/L	40–1400 mmol/kg
Typical urine	500–800 mOsm/L	500–800 mmol/kg
Urinary pH	4.5–8.0	4.5–8.0
Typical urine	<6.6	<6.6

(Source: Smeltzer, S. and Bare, B. (1996) Brunner and Suddarth's textbook of medical surgical nursing (8th ed.) Philadelphia: Lippincott-Raven.)

3. Blood is filtered through the glomerulus, and water and electrolytes enter the renal tubules.
4. The majority of electrolytes are reabsorbed in the proximal tubule, but reabsorption occurs along the entire length of the tubule.
   a. Tubular reabsorption can be compared with a sponge.
   b. Water is reabsorbed through specialized cells that line the tubules.
   c. The amount of water reabsorbed depends on the amount needed by the body.

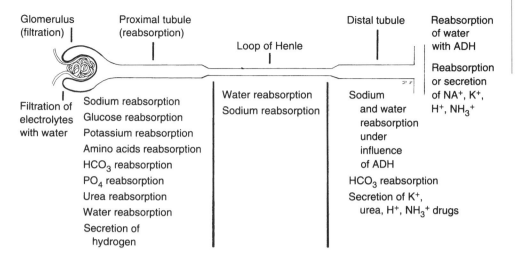

FIGURE 4-2.
Reabsorption and secretion of electrolytes along the kidney tubule.

    d. As water moves through the length of the tubule, less water is present for reabsorption at the distal ends than in the proximal ends.

    e. In the distal and collecting tubules, water is reabsorbed only in the presence of anti-diuretic hormone (which is released when the body needs more water).

    f. As water is reabsorbed through the length of the tubules, electrolytes are also reabsorbed.

    g. Electrolytes move from one side of the tubular membrane to the other in order to maintain electrical neutrality (Fig. 4-2).

  5. *Electrolyte secretion* occurs when an electrolyte moves from the blood into the tubule, as opposed to entering the tubule through glomerular filtration.

  6. Some electrolytes are regulated by secretion and reabsorption.

C. Endocrine regulation

  1. Along with the kidneys, the endocrine system is the primary regulator of electrolytes.

  2. Pituitary adrenocorticotropic hormone stimulation enhances adrenal release of aldosterone.

  3. Aldosterone acts on the tubules to reabsorb sodium.

  4. When sodium is reabsorbed, another positively charged electrolyte—the cation potassium—is secreted into the tubules for excretion.

D. Gastrointestinal regulation

  1. Electrolytes are secreted, absorbed, and exchanged across the bowel the same way they are in the kidney.

  2. Gastric juices are high in acid content, and the exchange between anions and cations occurs across the small bowel (Tables 1-1 and 1-2 and Figs. 4-1 and 4-2).

Bibliography

Bullock, B. (1996). *Pathophysiology: Adaptations and alterations in function* (4th ed.). Philadelphia: J. B. Lippincott.

Guyton, A. (1991). *Textbook of medical physiology* (8th ed.). Philadelphia: W. B. Saunders.

Kinney, M., Packa, D., & Dunbar, S. (1993). *AACN's clinical reference for critical-care nursing* (3rd ed.). St. Louis: C.V. Mosby.

Kokko, J., & Tannen, R. (1996). *Fluids and electrolytes* (3rd ed.). Philadelphia: W. B. Saunders.

Metheny, N. (1996). *Fluid and electrolyte balance: Nursing considerations* (3rd ed.). Philadelphia: J. B. Lippincott.

Miller, M. (1997). Fluid and electrolyte homeostasis in the elderly: physiologic changes of aging and clinical consequences. *Baillieres Clinical Endocrinology and Metabolism,* 11(2), 367–387.

Narrins, R. (Ed). (1994). *Maxwell & Kleemans clinical disorders of fluid and electrolyte metabolism* (5th ed.). New York: McGraw-Hill.

North American Nursing Diagnosis Association. Nursing Diagnosis: Definitions and Classifications. The Auth. 1996.

Plante, G. E., Chakir, M., Lehoux, S., & Lortie, M. (1995). Disorders of body fluid balance: A new look into the mechanisms of disease. *Canadian Journal of Cardiology.* 11(9), 788–802.

Porth, C. (1994). *Pathophysiology: Concepts of altered health states* (4th ed.). Philadelphia: J. B. Lippincott.

Rose, B. (1994). *Clinical physiology of acid-base and electrolyte disorders* (4th ed.). New York: McGraw-Hill.

Seaman, S. L. (1995). Renal physiology part II: Fluid and electrolyte regulation. *Neonatal network,* 14(5), 5–11.

Smith, K., & Brain, E. (1991). *Fluids and electrolytes: A conceptual approach* (2nd ed.). New York: Churchill Livingstone.

Szerlip, H., & Goldfarb, S. (1993). *Workshops in fluid and electrolyte disorders.* New York: Churchill Livingstone.

Toto, K. (1994). Endocrine physiology. *Critical Care Nursing Clinics of North America,* December, 647–657.

STUDY QUESTIONS

1. Electrolytes are responsible for all of the following functions *except:*
   a. maintaining the osmolality of body fluid compartments
   b. regulating the balance of acids and bases
   c. aiding in neurologic and neuromuscular conduction
   d. regulating body fluids

2. Major intracellular fluid (ICF) electrolytes include:
   a. sodium
   b. potassium
   c. chloride
   d. bicarbonate

3. Primary ACTH stimulation will result in:
   a. sodium reabsorption
   b. sodium excretion
   c. potassium reabsorption
   d. decreased aldosterone release

4. When caring for a patient who has had a small bowel resection and is 1-day postoperative, the nurse is aware that the patient is at risk for electrolyte imbalance because of:
   a. impaired nutrient intake
   b. impaired exchange between anions and cations
   c. pain
   d. impaired endocrine stimulation

5. Cations are defined as:
   a. positively charged ions
   b. negatively charged ions
   c. enzyme-like substances
   d. precursors of electrolytes

6. The chief cation found in the extracellular fluid (ECF) is:
   a. sodium
   b. potassium
   c. chloride
   d. phosphorus

7. Which of the following statements is true?
   a. ECF electrolytes are found within the cell membrane.
   b. ICF electrolytes are easily measurable.
   c. ICF electrolytes have a nonvariable concentration.
   d. ICF electrolyte values are inferred from ECF values.

8. Which of the following is a normal source of electrolyte intake?
   a. medications
   b. Gatorade
   c. IV solutions
   d. hyperalimentation

9. Which structure in the kidney is responsible for filtration of electrolytes:
   a. glomerulus
   b. proximal tubule
   c. loop of Henle
   d. distal tubule

10. The nurse caring for a patient who has lost a large volume of gastric fluid knows that the patient is also losing:
    a. bases
    b. acids
    c. water
    d. none of the above

ANSWER KEY

Question	Correct answer	Correct answer rationale	Incorrect answer rationales
1.	d	Electrolytes do not play a primary role in the regulation of body fluids.	a, b, and c. Electrolytes do main-body fluid osmolality, regulate the balance of acid and bases, and aid in neurologic conduction.
2.	b	Potassium is the major cation found in the ICF.	a, c, and d. Sodium, chloride, and bicarbonate are found in greater amounts in the ECF.
3.	a	Stimulation of ACTH will result in increased aldosterone release and, therefore, increased sodium reabsorption.	b. Sodium is reabsorbed, not excreted. c. Potassium will be excreted as sodium is reabsorbed. d. Aldosterone release is increased with ACTH.
4.	b	Gastrointestinal balance of electrolytes involves the exchange of cations and anions in the small bowel; surgery would interfere with this for a period of time.	a. Nutrient intake refers to the ability to eat. c. Pain does not alter electrolyte balance. d. There is no endocrine impairment associated with bowel surgery.
5.	a	Cations are positively charged ions.	b. Anions are negatively charged ions. c and d. These responses are not the definition of cations.
6.	a	Sodium is the primary cation found in the ECF.	b. Potassium is the chief cation of the ICF. c and d. These are anions.
7.	d	ICF electrolytes cannot be measured, and their values are inferred from extracellular values.	a. ECF electrolytes are found outside of the cell membrane. b and c. ICF electrolyte concentrations fluctuate based on normal and abnormal occurrences, and this compartment cannot be directly measured.
8.	b	Food and fluids like Gatorade are normal sources of electrolytes for humans.	a, c, and d. These are abnormal sources necessary for patients who experience electrolyte deficits.
9.	a	The glomerulus is responsible for filtration.	b, c, and d. These structures are are found along the convoluted renal tubules. These structures do not filter.
10.	b	Gastric juices are rich in acid molecules. Loss of gastric fluids often results in loss of acids.	a. Loss of bases is not associated with loss of gastric fluid. c. Loss of water is addressed in the stem.

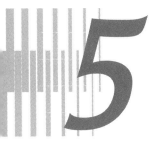

Sodium: Normal and Altered Balance

I. Normal balance

A. Description

1. Sodium is the major extracellular fluid (ECF) cation.
2. Normal serum sodium concentration ranges from 136 to 145 mEq/L.
3. Sodium is regulated proportionally with water and chloride.

B. Supply and sources

1. Most sodium is found outside of the cell in the ECF where it can be measured by serum tests.

2. **Some sodium is found in the intracellular fluid (ICF), but it is not measurable.**

3. Sodium is taken in through the diet. The minimum sodium requirement for adults is 2 g daily; most adults consume more because sodium is abundant in almost all foods.

C. Functions

1. Because sodium is found in abundance in the ECF, its balance is important for many physiologic functions, including:

    a.   Facilitating impulse transmission in nerve and muscle fibers by participating in the sodium-potassium pump

    b.   Influencing the levels of potassium and chloride by exchanging for potassium and attracting to chloride

    c.   Assisting in acid–base balance by combining with bicarbonate and chloride

2.   **Sodium also determines the volume and osmolality of the ECF and regulates body water.**

D.   **Regulation**

    1.   Sodium is lost through the skin, gastrointestinal tract, and genitourinary tract.

    2.   Renal and endocrine mechanisms contribute to sodium balance.

    3.   The kidneys match sodium excretion to sodium intake:

        a.   Through glomerular filtration, sodium passes through the glomerular filter along with water.

        b.   Through tubular reabsorption, sodium is reabsorbed with water along the course of the tubules, mostly in the proximal tubule. The presence of aldosterone in the tubules will enhance reabsorption of sodium.

    4.   The endocrine system secretes aldosterone and antidiuretic hormone (ADH) to help regulate sodium levels and maintain the balance between sodium and water:

        a.   When ECF sodium is decreased, the adrenal glands send aldosterone to the kidneys, where sodium is reabsorbed.

        b.   When ECF sodium is increased, aldosterone secretion is decreased, allowing sodium excretion.

        c.   When ECF sodium is elevated, ECF osmolality also is elevated, and ADH is secreted; this increases tubular reabsorption of water.

        d.   Decreased ECF sodium reduces ECF osmolality.

        e.   Pituitary secretion of adrenocorticotropin hormone helps regulate sodium by increasing the presence of aldosterone.

II.   Sodium deficiency: Hyponatremia

A.   **Description:** Serum sodium levels below 136 mEq/L

B.   **Etiology**

    1.   **Sodium loss in excess of water, which can result from:**

        a.   **Prolonged diuretic therapy (which impairs sodium reabsorption in Henle's loop)**

        b.   **Excessive burns (which cause a large loss of ECF, where sodium concentration is high)**

        c.   **Excessive diaphoresis (because sodium is found in large amounts in sweat)**

        d.   **Prolonged vomiting, nasogastric suction, diarrhea, or laxative abuse**

        e.   **Renal disease**

    2.   **Water gain in excess of sodium, which could result from:**

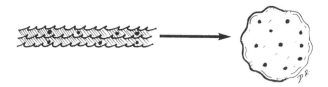

FIGURE 5-1.
Hyponatremia. When water is present in excess of sodium, water will move into the cell, causing it to swell.

  a. Excessive administration of water, as in intravenous solutions, such as D_5W; eventually water will shift into the ICF in an attempt to balance the ratio of sodium to water (Fig. 5-1).
  b. Compulsive water drinking that occurs with some psychiatric disorders; this results in diluted sodium levels and allows water to shift into the cells.
3. Inadequate intake or absorption, such as due to anorexia or acute alcoholism
4. Adrenal insufficiency, in which aldosterone levels are low and sodium reabsorption becomes compromised, thus allowing sodium excretion
5. Syndrome of inappropriate ADH (SIADH), in which water is retained and dilutional hyponatremia occurs

C. Assessment findings

 1. Clinical manifestations may include vomiting and diarrhea; however, these symptoms may actually be the cause of hyponatremia.

 2. Neurologic and musculoskeletal symptoms may occur because sodium is required for normal functioning of these systems; such symptoms may include:
  a. Muscle cramps
  b. Muscle twitching
  c. Headache
  d. Dizziness
  e. Confusion
  f. Convulsions
  g. Coma

3. Because sodium is required for regulation of ECF volume and balance of ECF water, water shifts from the ECF to the ICF, causing cells to swell and resulting in central nervous system (CNS) symptoms.
4. As sodium is lost, the serum becomes more concentrated. Laboratory tests reveal:
  a. Serum sodium level below 136 mEq/L
  b. Urine specific gravity > 1.010
  c. Serum osmolality > 285 mOsm/kg

D. Potential nursing diagnoses

1. Fluid Volume Excess
2. High Risk for Injury
3. Anxiety

    4. Fatigue
    5. Impaired Physical Mobility
    6. Activity Intolerance

E. Interventions

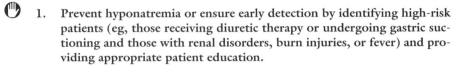 1. Prevent hyponatremia or ensure early detection by identifying high-risk patients (eg, those receiving diuretic therapy or undergoing gastric suctioning and those with renal disorders, burn injuries, or fever) and providing appropriate patient education.

2. Aid in the treatment objective of restoring serum sodium level.

3. Restrict water intake to allow sodium and water to balance naturally.

4. Administer hypertonic solutions (eg, 3% normal saline) *with extreme caution;* these solutions will force water to leave the ICF to balance the sodium instilled in the ECF, thus causing cellular shrinkage. The expansion of the extracellular space may cause excessive demands on the heart and lead to congestive heart failure.

5. Measure and record daily weights to track fluid retention and loss.

6. Monitor vital signs and serum sodium levels.

F. Evaluation

    1. Serum sodium level returns to a range between 136 and 145 mEq/L.
    2. The patient remains free of symptoms.

III. Sodium excess: Hypernatremia

A. Description: Serum sodium level above 145 mEq/L

B. Etiology

1. Sodium gain in excess of water, such as from:
    a. Administration of hypertonic parenteral solutions or tube feedings
    b. Excessive dietary intake of sodium, which may occur through the normal route or through parenteral and enteral feedings

2. Water loss in excess of sodium, such as from:
    a. Severe watery stool
    b. Severe insensible water loss
    c. Burns
    d. Osmotic diuresis
    e. Diabetes insipidus

3. Fluid shifts:
    a. In certain conditions, water will shift out of the ICF into the ECF to balance the excess ECF sodium.
    b. This causes the cells to shrink as they lose water volume (Fig. 5-2).

C. Assessment findings

    1. Symptoms of hypernatremia often are associated with those of dehydration, including:
        a. Thirst
        b. Tachycardia

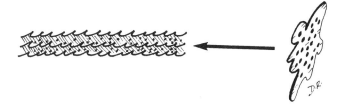

FIGURE 5-2.
Hypernatremia. When sodium is present in excess of water, water will move out of the cell, causing the cell to shrink.

    c. Dry mucous membranes
    d. Lethargy
  2. Because sodium is required for normal neurologic and musculoskeletal conduction, hypernatremia commonly has CNS manifestations, including:
    a. Hyperactive reflexes
    b. Lethargy
    c. Seizures
  3. As sodium is retained or fluid shifts, the serum becomes more dilute; laboratory tests reveal:
    a. Serum sodium level > 145 mEq/L
    b. Urine specific gravity > 1.015
    c. Serum osmolality > 295 mOsm/kg

D. **Potential nursing diagnoses**
  1. Fluid Volume Deficit
  2. High Risk for Injury
  3. Fatigue
  4. Altered Nutrition: Less Than Body Requirements

E. **Interventions**
  1. Identify high-risk patients (eg, those receiving hypertonic tube feedings or hypertonic total parenteral nutrition [TPN] solutions), and provide appropriate patient education.
  2. Aid in the treatment objective of reducing the serum sodium level.
  3. Measure and record daily weights to monitor fluid retention and loss.
  4. Record intake and output because the patient may have a markedly decreased output.
  5. Assess vital signs.
  6. Assess mentation.
  7. Administer parenteral solutions *with caution;* hypotonic sodium solutions—*except D_5W*—are best to prevent fluid overload.
  8. Monitor laboratory tests.
  9. Ensure adequate water intake if a patient is receiving hypertonic fluid to prevent solute overload (eg, dilute tube feedings and be sure to infuse TPN at prescribed rate).

F. **Evaluation**
  1. Serum sodium level returns to a range between 136 and 145 mEq/L.
  2. The patient remains free of symptoms.

Bibliography

Bullock, B. (1996). *Pathophysiology: Adaptations and alterations in function* (4th ed.). Philadelphia: J. B. Lippincott.

Drummer, C., Gerzer, R., Heer, M., et al. (1992). Effects of an acute saline infusion on fluid and electrolyte metabolism in humans. *American Journal of Physiology,* May, 744–754.

Guyton, A. (1991). *Textbook of medical physiology* (8th ed.). Philadelphia: W. B. Saunders.

Kinney, M., Packa, D., & Dunbar, S. (1993). *AACN's clinical reference for critical-care nursing* (3rd ed.). St. Louis: C.V. Mosby.

Kokko, J., & Tannen, R. (1996). *Fluids and electrolytes* (3rd ed.). Philadelphia: W. B. Saunders.

Metheny, N. (1996). *Fluid and electrolyte balance: Nursing considerations* (3rd ed.). Philadelphia: J. B. Lippincott.

Miller, M. (1997). Fluid and electrolyte homeostasis in the elderly: physiologic changes of aging and clinical consequences. *Baillieres Clinical Endocrinology and Metabolism,* 11(2), 367–387.

Narrins, R. (Ed). (1994). *Maxwell & Kleemans clinical disorders of fluid and electrolyte metabolism* (5th ed.). New York: McGraw-Hill.

North American Nursing Diagnosis Association. Nursing Diagnosis: Definitions and Classifications. The Auth. 1996.

Plante, G. E., Chakir, M., Lehoux, S., & Lortie, M. (1995). Disorders of body fluid balance: A new look into the mechanisms of disease. *Canadian Journal of Cardiology,* 11(9), 788–802.

Porth, C. (1994). *Pathophysiology: Concepts of altered health states* (4th ed.). Philadelphia: J. B. Lippincott.

Rose, B. (1994). *Clinical physiology of acid-base and electrolyte disorders* (4th ed.). New York: McGraw-Hill.

Seaman, S. L. (1995). Renal physiology part II: Fluid and electrolyte regulation. *Neonatal network,* 14(5), 5–11.

Smith, K., & Brain, E. (1991). *Fluids and electrolytes: A conceptual approach* (2nd ed.). New York: Churchill Livingstone.

Szerlip, H., & Goldfarb, S. (1993). *Workshops in fluid and electrolyte disorders.* New York: Churchill Livingstone.

Toto, K. (1994). Endocrine physiology. *Critical Care Nursing Clinics of North America,* December, 647–657.

STUDY QUESTIONS

1. When assessing a patient for hypernatremia, the nurse would expect to find:
   a. serum sodium level of 135 mEq/L
   b. moist mucous membranes
   c. thirst
   d. hypoactive reflexes

2. Which of the following IV solutions would the nurse administer for a patient with hypernatremia?
   a. 3% saline
   b. 0.33% saline
   c. D₅W
   d. lactated Ringer's solution

3. When ECF sodium is decreased, the adrenal glands send aldosterone to the kidneys to:
   a. increase sodium reabsorption
   b. decrease sodium reabsorption
   c. increase water reabsorption
   d. decrease water reabsorption

4. Patients at high risk for hyponatremia include:
   a. patients receiving hypotonic TPN
   b. patients on diuretic therapy
   c. burn victims
   d. patients with gastric suctioning

5. The nurse should administer hypertonic IV solutions with caution because these solutions will force:
   a. water to leave the ECF
   b. water to leave the ICF
   c. cellular swelling
   d. hydrostatic pressure to drop

6. Aldosterone reabsorption of sodium occurs after stimulation with:
   a. Adrenocorticotropic hormone (ACTH)
   b. insulin
   c. antidiuretic hormone (ADH)
   d. pitocin

7. When caring for a patient with hyponatremia, the nurse is careful to restrict:
   a. water
   b. sodium
   c. potassium
   d. chloride

8. When caring for a patient with hypernatremia, the nurse is careful to administer:
   a. water
   b. sodium
   c. potassium
   d. chloride

9. Which electrolyte imbalance will cause cellular shrinking:
   a. hypernatremia
   b. hyponatremia
   c. hyperkalemia
   d. hypokalemia

10. The danger of hyponatremia is:
    a. neurologic effects
    b. cardiac effects
    c. renal response
    d. blood gas changes

ANSWER KEY

Question	Correct answer	Correct answer rationale	Incorrect answer rationales
1.	c	Thirst and other signs of dehydration indicate hypernatremia.	a. Serum sodium level is greater than 145 mEq/L in hypernatremia. b. Dry, not moist mucous membranes are found in hypernatremia. c. Reflexes are hyperactive, not hypoactive in hypernatremia.
2.	b	Hypotonic solutions are prescribed for a patient with hypernatremia; 0.33% saline is hypotonic.	b. 3% saline solution is hypertonic. c. D_5W is contraindicated because of the possibility of fluid overload. d. This response is isotonic.
3.	a	When ECF sodium is decreased, the adrenal glands send aldosterone to the kidneys to increase sodium reabsorption in an attempt to to balance sodium levels.	b, c, and d. These responses are incorrect.
4.	b	Patients on diuretics may develop hyponatremia as sodium is lost in excess of water.	a. Patients receiving hypertonic TPN are at risk to develop hypernatremiac, and c and d. Cardiac and renal diseases are not necessarily a cause of hyponatremia.
5.	b	Hypertonic IV fluids will force water to leave the ICF to balance the sodium in the ECF, thus causing cell shrinkage.	a, c and d. These responses are incorrect.
6.	a	Adrenocorticotropic hormone (ACTH) is released from the pituitary; it stimulates adrenal release of aldosterone.	b, c, and d. These do not influence sodium reabsorption.
7.	a	In hyponatremia, water is present in excessive amounts.	b, c, and d. These are electrolyte replacements and are not suitable treatment choices for hyponatremia.
8.	a	Patients with hypernatremia are thirsty; they need water replacement to balance the rising sodium levels.	b, c, and d. These are not appropriate treatments for hypernatremia.
9.	a	Hypernatremia causes cellular shrinking.	b, c, and d. These imbalances do not cause cellular shrinking.
10.	a	Hyponatremia has adverse effects on the central nervous system as the cells of the brain become "waterlogged."	b, c, and d. These responses are not dangers associated with hyponatremia.

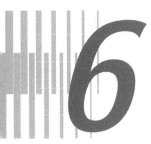

6 Potassium: Normal and Altered Balance

I. Normal balance

A. Description
   1. Potassium is the major cation in intracellular fluid (ICF).
   2. Normal serum potassium concentration ranges from 3.5 to 5.0 mEq/L.

B. Supply and sources
   1. Potassium is taken in through the diet; it is found abundantly in citrus fruits, vegetables, chocolate, and licorice.
   2. Abnormal routes of potassium intake include intravenous (IV) solutions and nutritional supplements.
   3. Potassium is lost from the gastrointestinal (GI) and renal systems.
   4. Abnormal amounts of potassium are lost through the excess elimination of urine and stool.
   5. Ninety-eight percent of all potassium is found inside the cell; 2% is found in extracellular fluid (ECF). This 2% is reflected in serum concentration measurements.

   6. *Important:* **When measuring serum potassium, the result reflects only 2%. The result can represent a shift of the electrolyte from one compartment to another, *or* a rapid gain/loss depending on the situation.**

C.   **Functions**

1. Because potassium is positively charged and is found in the ICF, its balance is important for several physiologic functions, including:
   a. Regulating osmolarity of ECF by exchanging with sodium
   b. Maintaining the transmembrane electrical potential that exists between the ICF and ECF
   c. Maintaining normal neuromuscular contraction by participation in the sodium-potassium pump
   d. Maintaining *all* muscular activity—with a particular sensitivity to cardiac muscle—through its role in the sodium-potassium pump
2. Along with sodium, potassium maintains acid–base balance as it exchanges for hydrogen.
3. Potassium is required for all metabolic processes, including:
   a. Carbohydrate metabolism
   b. Glycogen synthesis
   c. Protein synthesis

D.   **Regulation**

1. Potassium is regulated by:
   a. Renal mechanisms
   b. Extrarenal mechanisms
2. *Renal mechanisms* include:
   a. Glomerular filtration
   b. Tubular reabsorption
   c. Tubular secretion
   d. Renin-aldosterone mechanism
   e. Plasma protein regulation
   f. Sodium regulation
   g. Metabolic acidosis
3. In *glomerular filtration,* blood is filtered in the glomerulus, where the filtered load enters the proximal tubule.
4. In *tubular reabsorption:*
   a. The epithelial cells of the proximal tubule reabsorb approximately 65% of the filtered potassium through active transport.
   b. The thick portion of the ascending limb of Henle's loop reabsorbs about 27%, leaving 8% of the original filtered load to enter the distal tubules.
   c. The distal and collecting tubules absorb a very slight amount of potassium, but potassium secretion occurs here.
5. In *tubular secretion,* potassium moves from the blood to the tubular lumen:
   a. The amount of potassium secretion is determined by the need for potassium elimination, which is influenced by the serum concentration level.
   b. Potassium is exchanged for hydrogen to maintain electrical neutrality across the cell membrane.
   c. Because potassium and sodium must exchange for balance, the sodium concentration and the presence of aldosterone will increase

absorption of sodium from the tubules to the serum, making potassium exchange the other way (eg, be excreted) to achieve balance.

6. The distal tubule's secretory function provides evidence of why hyperkalemia is consistent with tubular defects seen in various forms of acute and chronic renal failure.

7. During end-stage renal disease, glomerular filtration or tubular reabsorption and secretion fail.

8. The *renin-aldosterone mechanism,* which is mediated by angiotensin, brings a supply of aldosterone to the distal tubule and affects potassium levels:

   a. Aldosterone in the tubule causes reabsorption of sodium, which in turn causes potassium to move in the opposite direction from the blood into the tubule for secretions.

   b. Aldosterone also stimulates potassium uptake in the proximal tubule, increasing the concentration of peritubular potassium. This enhances passive diffusion of potassium into the tubular lumen for excretion when it arrives in the distal tubule. This mechanism is targeted during administration of certain medications, such as Aldactone.

9. *Plasma protein* levels regulate potassium because an increase in plasma protein concentration causes a subsequent rise in the rate of potassium transport into the tubular lumen. This results from an increase in ICF electrical negativity that pulls potassium into the tubular cells and then into the tubular lumen.

10. *Sodium regulation* affects potassium levels:

    a. When the amount of sodium entering the distal tubule increases, the rate of sodium reabsorption by the distal end of the tubules and collecting ducts also increases.

    b. As a result, potassium secretion, which normally moves in the opposite direction of sodium reabsorption by the distal end of the tubules and collecting ducts, also is increased.

    c. The sodium delivery to the distal tubule fosters potassium secretion by increasing the transmembrane electrical difference.

    d. Situations that contribute to natriuresis (sodium elimination) increase potassium elimination and increase the osmotic load that exists when a large water supply is present.

    e. The larger the osmotic load delivered to the proximal tubule, the less potassium reabsorbed at this point, which makes more available for elimination.

11. *Metabolic acidosis* affects potassium levels as it is exchanged for hydrogen:

    a. During metabolic acidosis, hydrogen levels rise, then hydrogen moves to the ICF and potassium moves out of the ICF to restore electrical neutrality.

    b. As a result, the ICF concentration of potassium in the distal tubule is diminished.

    c. Additional bicarbonate wasting provides accelerated distal delivery of the anion, increasing potassium secretion in another attempt to maintain electrical neutrality.

12. *Extrarenal mechanisms* that affect potassium regulation include:

    a. GI system

         b.   Fluid shifts

         c.   Hydration

13.   In the *GI system,* the mucosa of the large bowel is readily responsive to some of the same stimulators of kaliuresis (potassium excretion):

         a.   Mineralocorticoid activity causes sodium reabsorption and potassium elimination from the same mechanism that occurs in the kidney.

         b.   Accelerated bowel elimination of potassium is an important adaptive mechanism. (For this reason, patients undergoing bowel surgery or those with large amounts of GI drainage must be watched closely for dropping potassium levels.)

14.   Potassium levels are sensitive to hormonal fluctuations and any conditions that could cause *fluid shifts,* including:

         a.   Adrenocorticotropic hormone (ACTH) secretion: ACTH is secreted from the anterior pituitary to stimulate steroid secretion from the adrenal glands, making aldosterone levels dependent on ACTH levels. In the presence of aldosterone, sodium is retained and potassium is excreted. Potassium levels drop when ACTH levels rise due to the relationship between ACTH and aldosterone. Potassium levels rise as ACTH and aldosterone levels drop, because sodium is eliminated rather than reabsorbed.

         b.   Increased glucose levels: As glucose levels rise, potassium is transported into the cells. As glucose levels drop, potassium leaves the cell.

15.   *Hydration* affects potassium levels in two ways:

         a.   Increased body water (hypervolemia) can dilute potassium, causing levels to drop.

         b.   Dehydration (hypovolemia) causes an increase in potassium concentration, resulting in higher serum levels.

II.   Potassium deficiency: Hypokalemia

A.   Description: Serum potassium level below 3.5 mEq/L

B.   Etiology

1.   **Potassium loss, such as from:**

         a.   **Prolonged diuretic therapy (because potassium follows water and sodium across the tubular membrane)**

         b.   **Prolonged vomiting, diarrhea, laxative abuse, or nasogastric suctioning (because bile and GI secretions are rich in potassium) causes severe GI losses.**

         c.   **Severe diaphoresis**

         d.   **Renal tubule defects (occur with various renal diseases)**

         e.   **Excessive removal of potassium during peritoneal dialysis or hemodialysis**

2.   Inadequate intake or absorption due to:

         a.   Anorexia

         b.   Acute alcoholism

3.   Fluid and electrolyte shifts due to:

         a.   Administration of potassium-deficient hyperalimentation solutions

      b. Administration of hypertonic glucose solutions (because potassium may shift from ECF to ICF)

      c. Presence of excessive amounts of exogenous or endogenous insulin (because insulin acts as a carrier molecule, aiding intracellular transport of potassium)

      d. Presence of excessive steroid hormones (because corticosteroid levels influence sodium retention and reciprocal potassium excretion)

      e. Lowered levels of extracellular hydrogen (such as occurs in metabolic alkalosis)

      f. Hyperaldosteronism (which causes excessive absorption of sodium in the proximal tubules, accounting for accelerated excretion of potassium)

C. Assessment findings

  1. Clinical manifestations may include vomiting or diarrhea; however, these symptoms may be the cause of hypokalemia.

  2. Because potassium is required for normal musculoskeletal contractions, alterations will affect the musculoskeletal system. Symptoms may include:

      a. Muscle weakness and cramps

      b. Hyporeflexia

      c. Paresthesias

      d. Decreased bowel motility (which could develop into paralytic ileus)

      e. Hypotension

      f. Cardiac dysrhythmia

      g. Drowsiness, lethargy, coma

  3. Laboratory results reveal:

      a. Serum potassium level below 3.5 mEq/L

      b. pH elevated above 7.45

      c. Decreased serum bicarbonate level

      d. Elevated glucose level (possible)

  4. **Another diagnostic cue is electrocardiogram (EKG) changes; as potassium levels drop, the EKG will gradually reveal ST segment depression, flattened T waves, and U waves that may be hidden on the T waves (Fig. 6-1).**

D. Potential nursing diagnoses

  1. Decreased Cardiac Output

  2. High Risk for Injury

  3. Anxiety

  4. Altered Nutrition: Less Than Body Requirements

  5. Impaired Physical Mobility

  6. Activity Intolerance

E. Interventions

  1. Prevent hypokalemia and ensure early detection by identifying high-risk patients (eg, those who have anorexia, diarrhea, or nausea and vomiting) and providing appropriate patient education.

  2. Teach patients receiving diuretic therapy at home about hypokalemia and how to manage it.

  3. Be aware that in patients receiving digitalis, digitalis toxicity may occur (especially if Lasix is administered concurrently).

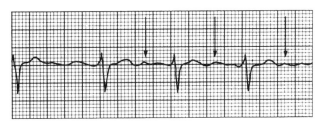

A

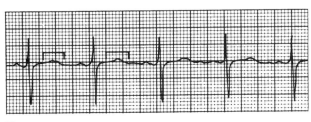

B

FIGURE 6-1.
(A) Presence of U waves (hypokalemia). **(B)** Fusion of T and U waves (hypokalemia).

4. Monitor intake and output, keeping in mind that urine contains potassium.
5. Replace potassium through dietary intervention (eg, encourage the patient to eat or drink citrus fruits and juices).
6. Administer oral potassium replacements, as ordered; be aware that these can irritate the GI mucosa, so give them with water. Display 6-1 describes the nurse's implications when administering potassium supplements.
7. When adding potassium to a liter of IV solution:
    a. Be sure the drip rate is adjusted so that replacement does not occur too quickly.
    b. Be aware that the insertion site may become reddened and painfully irritated.
    c. Be sure to mix the solution thoroughly, or the patient may inadvertently receive a potassium bolus.
    d. Keep in mind that rapid administration of potassium can cause sudden hyperkalemia, which can cause cardiac arrest.
8. **For life-threatening hypokalemia:**
    a. **Replace potassium more rapidly by adding 10 mEq of potassium chloride to 100 mL of IV solution and infusing over 1 hour using an infusion pump.**
    b. **Use *extreme caution*, and *never administer potassium by IV push method*, which could cause death.**
    c. Institute cardiac monitoring. Display 6-2 describes concepts necessary for the nurse to understand in order to safely administer potassium replacement.
9. Monitor vital signs.

DISPLAY 6-1
Nursing Considerations in Administering Oral Potassium Supplements

1. The most common adverse reactions to oral potassium salts are nausea, vomiting, abdominal discomfort, and diarrhea. To help minimize GI irritation, administer potassium supplements immediately after meals or with food.
2. Hyperkalemia can result from oral overdosage, just as it can from intravenous overdosage. Therefore, care should be taken to administer the intended dose. Because there are numerous forms of potassium supplements available commercially, with highly variable concentrations, it is important to check the physician's order carefully against the preparation's label (some trade names are quite similar).
3. A single oral dose of potassium should probably not exceed the hourly intravenous dose (used in more life-threatening situations). The ingestion of more than 160 mEq can reduce a potentially fatal increase in the serum potassium concentration to >8.0 mEq/L even when normal renal functiuon is present.
4. Potassium supplements are contraindicated in patients receiving potassium-sparing diuretics (ie, spironolactone [Aldactone], triameterene [Dyrenium], and amiloride [Midamor]).
5. Dosages of potassium supplements need to be decreased (or perhaps even discontinued) if the patient begins to use generous portions of potassium-containing salt substitutes.
6. Slow-release tablets should be administered with a full glass of water to help them dissolve in the GI tract. Observe patients taking slow-release KCl tablets for GI bleeding as these tablets may cause intestinal and gastric ulceration. Do not crush potassium tablets unless the manufacturer's directions specifically state that it is appropriate.
7. Effervescent potassium supplements should be dissolved in 3 to 8 oz cold water, juice or suitable beverage and consumed slowly.
8. The majority of patients with hypokalemia have mild to moderate decreases in serum potassium levels (such as 3.0–3.5 mEq/L); this range is usually well tolerated in the absence of digitalis therapy or severe hepatic disease. Provided they can swallow, these patients can usually be treated with oral potassium supplements in the range of 60–80 mEq/L.

(Source: Metheny, N. M. (1996). Fluid and electrolyte balance (3rd ed.). Philadelphia: Lippincott-Raven.)

    10.   Monitor serum potassium levels.

    11.   Monitor for signs of other associated electrolyte disorders (eg, alkalosis).

F.   **Evaluation**

    1.   Serum potassium level returns to a range between 3.5 and 5.0 mEq/L.

    2.   The patient's cardiac output is normal.

    3.   The patient is free from injury.

III.   **Potassium excess: Hyperkalemia**

A.   **Description: Serum potassium level above 5.0 mEq/L**

B.   **Etiology**

    1.   Potassium intake in excess of potassium excretion, such as from:

        a.   IV replacement potassium

        b.   Potassium-rich hyperalimentation solutions

        c.   Use of potassium replacements

        d.   Excessive use of salt substitutes

DISPLAY 6-2
Nursing Considerations in Administering Potassium Intravenously

1. Concentrated potassium solutions from ampules should never be administered without first being diluted appropriately.

   Because of reports of deaths caused by the accidental injection of undiluted potassium chloride injections, the United States Pharmacopeia (USP) recently renamed the drug "potassium chloride for injection concentrate." To decrease the likelihood of mistaking the concentrate for a ready-to-use solution, the caps and overseals bear the words "must be diluted" and black bands with the words "must be diluted" appear on ampules (effective January 15, 1993). Furthermore, in order to minimize errors, many hospitals have removed potassium chloride for injection concentrate from nursing units and replaced it with minibags of potassium chloride injection 20 mEq/100 ml. The rationale is that if that form of the drug is administered in error, it is not likely to seriously harm anyone.

2. The appropriate dilution of potassium chloride solutions depends on (a) the amount of fluid the patient can tolerate, (b) the site of administration (peripheral or central vein), and (c) the patient's tolerance for pain at the infusion site.

Fluid Tolerance

It is safer to dilute potassium to the maximal point allowed without exceeding the patient's tolerance for fluid. For example, if a patient requires 80 mEq of KCl in 24 hr, and the fluid intake for that period is 2000 mL, the 80 mEq of KCl should be divided equally between the 2 L of allowable fluid (that is, 40 mEq/L). However, if a patient requires more potassium than can be administered at "typical" dilutions, it becomes necessary to administer more concentrated solutions. See below.

Site

Peripheral Vein. A typical concentration of potassium for peripheral veins is 20 to 40 mEq/L. The most frequently recommended maximal concentration of KCl in a peripheral vein is 60 mEq/L because higher concentrations are very irritating, resulting in pain and sclerosis of veins.

Central Vein. The maximal recommended concentration in a central vein is variable defined as 140 mEq/L (14 mEq/100 mL) to 200 mEq/L (20 mEq/100 mL). Unlike peripheral veins, central veins have a large blood flow, thereby allowing dilution of the irritating potassium solution. Although some authors have expressed concern that administering concentrated potassium solutions through central veins near the myocardium could cause dysrhythmias, this was not shown to be a problem in a study of 495 sets of KCl infusions administered to a population in a medical intensive care unit.

Tolerance for Pain at Infusion Site

Administration of KCl in a peripheral vein at a concentration >40 mEq/L is often associated with discomfort that increases as the concentration of KCl increases. Pain is more likely if the patient already has phlebitis associated with prolonged intravenous cannulation at the site and other irritating medications are also administered. The following steps are helpful in minimizing pain associated with the administration of KCl solutions:

(A) Dilute the KCl as much as possible.

(B) If a central line is in place, consider using this site for the infusion because rapid blood flow will dilute the KCl solution.

(C) If necessary, discuss with the physician the use of a small volume of lidocaine (either as a bolus through the IV device before the infusion or added to the solution) to minimize pain. Several studies have indicated that this method is of some benefit in alleviating pain associated with concentrated KCl solutions in peripheral veins:

> In a double-blind study of 28 subjects, researchers evaluated the effectiveness of a pretreatment IV bolus dose of 3 mL of lignocaine (versus a placebo bolus dose of 3 mL of 0.9% NaCl) at the infusion site in alleviating pain associated with the administration of concentrated KCl solutions (20 mEq/100 mL) over a 2-hr period. They concluded that pain at the IV site was significantly reduced in the group that received the lignocaine bolus dose.
>
> In an earlier study, the effect of lidocaine in alleviating pain induced by intravenous KCl

administration was evaluated in six healthy volunteers. Each subject received KCl in a concentration of 200 mEq/L (10 mEq of KCl in 50 mL D_5W) in both arms. One of the infusions had 10 mg of lidocaine added (although the subject was not told which infusion contained the lidocaine). The solutions were infused over 1 hr and each person was asked to rate the degree of pain in each arm on a 7-point scale (1 = mild, 7 = severe). It was found that pain was significantly less in the arm with the lidocaine (mean, 3.17) than in the arm without lidocaine (mean, 6.17). It is worth noting, however, that pain was still at least moderate in the group receiving the lidocaine.

3. Rate of administration is dependent on the urgency for potassium replacement:

    In usual situations, potassium is administered at a rate not exceeding 10 mEq/hr. In the presence of mild to moderate hypokalemia, it is safer to administer potassium at a rate no faster than 10–20 mEq/hr. Rates greater than 40 mEq/hr are not recommended because of the possibility of producing transient hyperkalemia and arrhythmias. However, as much as 40 to 100 mEq/hr have reportedly been given to patients with paralysis or life-threatening arrhythmias. Rapid potassium administration is potentially dangerous even in severely potassium-depleted patients and should be used only in life-threatening situations—ECG monitoring is essential in this setting.

4. Because potassium is primarily eliminated through the kidneys, it is important to monitor carefully the rate of urinary output. When giving potassium, a urine output >30 mL/hr is recommended to avoid producing transient hyperkalemia. If potassium replacement is needed in oliguric patients, the amount is reduced according to the level of renal function.

5. Because dextrose administered concurrently with potassium can cause a transient shift of potassium into the cells, urgent potassium replacement for severely hypokalemic patients is usually accomplished with a nondextrose solution (such as 0.9% sodium chloride solution).

6. Protocols for the safe administration of potassium solutions in specific institutions/agencies should be jointly written by nurses, physicians, and pharmacists. Such protocols are immensely helpful in preventing problems with potassium infusions. General precautions include:

    (A) Limit the amount of potassium available in a single container (such as 20 mEq in 100 mL of solution) to avoid accidental overinfusion.

    (B) Use an infusion pump to control the flow rate, and carefully monitor the rate to be sure that the pump doesn't malfunction. (Also, remember that KCl inadvertently administered into subcutaneous tissue is extremely injurious and needs to be detected early; pumps will continue to infuse KCl, regardless of whether the cannula is in the vein or subcutaneous tissue).

    (C) Mix KCl solutions with great care. Preferably, KCl solutions should be mixed in the pharmacy. If required to mix these solutions on a nursing unit, squeeze the medicine ports of plastic containers while they are in the upright position and then mix by inversion and agitation. Never add KCl to a hanging container (this can result in a high concentration bolus of the drug being administered). Commercially available premixed potassium-containing solutions are available in commonly prescribed concentrations for routine infusions.

(Source: Metheny, N. M. (1996). *Fluid and electrolyte balance* (3rd ed.). Philadelphia: Lippincott-Raven.)

2. Poor potassium elimination due to:
    a. Kidney failure (in which the tubules are unable to balance potassium)
    b. Bowel obstruction
    c. Use of potassium-sparing diuretics (spironolactone)
3. Electrolyte shifts in which a cation must leave the intracellular space, such as in:
    a. Metabolic acidosis: Hydrogen enters the cell in exchange for potassium, which leaves the cell and enters the ECF.
    b. Hyponatremia: When sodium is lost, potassium will move in the opposite direction and be retained.
4. **Cell lysis: In burns, trauma, cancer chemotherapy, or any condition causing great cell damage, potassium is released into the serum.**
5. Display 6-3 summarizes the etiologies of hyperkalemia.

C. **Assessment findings**
    1. Symptoms of hyperkalemia may be life-threatening.
    2. Because potassium is required for normal nerve and muscle contractions,

DISPLAY 6-3
Summary of Hyperkalemia

ETIOLOGICAL FACTORS	DEFINING CHARACTERISTICS
Pseudohyperkalemia	*Neuromuscular Effects*
• Prolonged tight application of tourniquet; fist clenching and unclenching immediately before or during blood drawing	• Vague muscular weakness
• Hemolysis of blood sample	• Flaccid muscle paralysis (first noticed in legs, later in arms and trunk; respiratory muscles and muscles supplied by cranial nerves are usually spared)
• Leukocytosis	
• Thrombocytosis	• Paresthesias of face, tongue, feet, and hands
Decreased Potassium Excretion	*Cardiovascular System*
• Oliguric renal failure	• Tall, peaked T waves
• Potassium-conserving diuretics	• Widened QRS complex progressing to sine waves
• Hypoaldosteronism	
High Potassium Intake	• Ventricular arrhythmias
• Improper use of oral potassium supplements	• Cardiac arrest
• Excessive use of salt substitutes	*Gastrointestinal System*
• Rapid intravenous potassium administration	• Nausea
• Rapid transfusion of aged blood	• Intermittent intestinal colic or diarrhea
Shift of Potassium out of Cells	*Laboratory Data*
• Acidosis	• Serum potassium >5.0 mEq/L
• Tissue damage, as in crushing injuries	• Often associated with acidosis
• Malignant cell lysis after chemotherapy	

(Metheny, N. M. (1996). Fluid and electrolyte balance (3rd ed.). Philadelphia: Lippincott-Raven)

hyperkalemia affects the musculoskeletal system, smooth muscle function, and nerve cell function; symptoms may include:
    a. Confusion
    b. Paresthesia
    c. Abdominal cramps with possible diarrhea
    d. Muscle paralysis
3. Because potassium is required for normal cardiac functioning, patients with hyperkalemia may present with life-threatening arrhythmias. As potassium levels rise, EKG changes worsen and include prolonged P-R interval, wide QRS complex, and full T waves (which may be tented). Eventually, these changes lead to cardiac arrest (Fig. 6-2).

D. Potential nursing diagnoses
    1. Decreased Cardiac Output
    2. High Risk for Injury
    3. Impaired Physical Mobility
    4. High Risk for Injury
    5. Pain
    6. Anxiety

E. Interventions

1. **Identify high-risk patients (eg, those receiving potassium-sparing diuretics, potassium supplements, or IV potassium and those with renal failure and metabolic acidosis).**
2. Check the patient's urine output and potassium levels before administering any medication containing potassium.
3. Provide cardiac monitoring.
4. If hyperkalemia is excessive, prepare the patient for either administration of Kayexelate, a glucose and insulin drip, or hemodialysis.
5. Administer sodium bicarbonate if ordered; be sure to administer this *with caution* because it can cause calcium levels to drop.
6. Monitor intake and output.

F. Evaluation
    1. Serum potassium level returns to a range between 3.5 and 5.0 mEq/L.

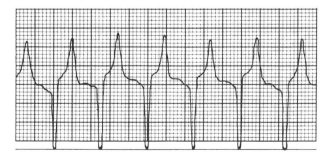

FIGURE 6-2.
Hyperkalemia and the presence of peaked T waves.

2. The patient remains free of symptoms.
3. Cardiac output is not decreased.
4. The patient is mobile and free from injury.

Bibliography

Bullock, B. (1996). *Pathophysiology: Adaptations and alterations in function* (4th ed.). Philadelphia: J. B. Lippincott.

Drummer, C., Gerzer, R., Heer, M., et al. (1992). Effects of an acute saline infusion on fluid and electrolyte metabolism in humans. *American Journal of Physiology,* May, 744–754.

Guyton, A. (1991). *Textbook of medical physiology.* (8th ed.). Philadelphia: W. B. Saunders.

Kinney, M., Packa, D., & Dunbar, S. (1993). *AACN's clinical reference for critical-care nursing* (3rd ed.). St. Louis: C.V. Mosby.

Kokko, J., & Tannen, R. (1996). *Fluids and electrolytes* (3rd ed.). Philadelphia: W. B. Saunders.

Metheny, N. (1996). *Fluid and electrolyte balance: Nursing considerations* (3rd ed.). Philadelphia: J. B. Lippincott.

Miller, M. (1997). Fluid and electrolyte homeostasis in the elderly: physiologic changes of aging and clinical consequences. *Baillieres Clinical Endocrinology and Metabolism,* 11(2), 367–387.

Narrins, R. (Ed). (1994). *Maxwell & Kleemans clinical disorders of fluid and electrolyte metabolism* (5th ed.). New York: McGraw-Hill.

North American Nursing Diagnosis Association. Nursing Diagnosis: Definitions and Classifications. The Auth. 1996.

Plante, G. E., Chakir, M., Lehoux, S., & Lortie, M. (1995). Disorders of body fluid balance: A new look into the mechanisms of disease. *Canadian Journal of Cardiology,* 11(9), 788–802.

Porth, C. (1994). *Pathophysiology: Concepts of altered health states* (4th ed.). Philadelphia: J. B. Lippincott.

Rose, B. (1994). *Clinical physiology of acid-base and electrolyte disorders* (4th ed.). New York: McGraw-Hill.

Seaman, S. L. (1995). Renal physiology part II: Fluid and electrolyte regulation. *Neonatal network,* 14(5), 5–11.

Smith, K., & Brain, E. (1991). *Fluids and electrolytes: A conceptual approach* (2nd ed.). New York: Churchill Livingstone.

Szerlip, H., & Goldfarb, S. (1993). *Workshops in fluid and electrolyte disorders.* New York: Churchill Livingstone.

Toto, K. (1994). Endocrine physiology. *Critical Care Nursing Clinics of North America,* December, 647–657.

STUDY QUESTIONS

1. When assessing a patient for potassium deficits, the nurse is aware that normal serum potassium level ranges from:
   a. 1.5 to 3.5 mEq/dl
   b. 2.5 to 4.5 mEq/dl
   c. 3.5 to 5.0 mEq/dl
   d. 4.0 to 7.5 mEq/dl

2. A patient who is on Lasix therapy asks the nurse about potassium-rich foods; which of the following foods would the nurse recommend?
   a. oranges
   b. apples
   c. pears
   d. peaches

3. Which of the following interventions would the nurse undertake for a patient receiving IV replacement of potassium?
   a. Assess level of consciousness.
   b. Monitor pulse.
   c. Monitor blood pressure.
   d. Assess the IV site.

4. Conditions that increase natriuresis result in:
   a. increased osmotic load and increased potassium excretion
   b. decreased osmotic load and decreased potassium excretion
   c. increased osmotic load and decreased potassium excretion
   d. decreased osmotic load and increased potassium excretion

5. Which of the following symptoms is not associated with hypokalemia?
   a. muscle cramps
   b. U waves on EKG
   c. paresthesia
   d. hyperreflexia

6. When assessing a patient for hyperkalemia, the nurse would expect to assess:

   a. V waves on EKG
   b. paresthesia
   c. decreased salivation
   d. tented P waves on EKG

7. Before administering any medication containing potassium, an important nursing intervention is to check the patient's:
   a. EKG
   b. pulse
   c. blood pressure
   d. urine output

8. Metabolic acidosis results in which of the following electrolyte shifts?
   a. Hydrogen ions are excreted with potassium and sodium.
   b. Hydrogen ions enter the ECF and potassium moves to the ICF.
   c. Hydrogen ions enter the cells and potassium moves to the ECF.
   d. Bicarbonate enters the cells in exchange for potassium ions.

9. When treating hyperkalemia, the physician prescribes sodium bicarbonate. Which may result from this administration:
   a. hypercalcemia
   b. hypocalcemia
   c. hypernatremia
   d. hyponatremia

10. Which may cause an intracellular shift of potassium:
   a. hypoaldosteronism
   b. steroid deficiency
   c. potassium rich TPN
   d. hypertonic glucose

ANSWER KEY

Question	Correct answer	Correct answer rationale	Incorrect answer rationales
1.	c	Normal serum potassium level ranges from 3.5 to 5.0 mEq/dl.	a, b, and d. Serum potassium level below 3.5 is hypokalemia; above 5.0, hyperkalemia.
2.	a	Citrus fruits, vegetables, chocolate, and licorice are good sources of potassium.	b, c, and d. These foods are not rich in potassium.
3.	d	Potassium supplements are irritating, so careful IV site assessment is necessary.	a, b, and c. These interventions are not related to IV administration of potassium.
4.	a	Conditions associated with natriuresis increase osmotic load and potassium excretion.	b, c, and d. These responses do not cause natriuresis.
5.	d	Hyporeflexia, not hyperreflexia, is a symptom of hypokalemia.	a, b, and c. Muscle cramps, U waves on the EKG, and paresthesia are additional symptoms of hypokalemia.
6.	b	Paresthesia is a sign of hyperkalemia.	a. There is no such wave known as a V wave. c. Salivation is not effected by potassium levels. d. The T wave, not the P wave is tented in hyperkalemia.
7.	d	Since kidney failure is an etiology of hyperkalemia, it is important that the nurse determine the patient's urine output before administering medications containing potassium.	a, b, and c. These are important parameters to assess, but are not specific to potassium.
8.	c	In metabolic acidosis, hydrogen ions enter the cells in exchange for potassium, which then leaves the cells and enters the ECF.	a, b, and d. These are electrolyte shifts that are not associated with metabolic acidosis.
9.	b	Administration of sodium bicarbonate can cause hypocalcemia.	a, c, and d. These alterations are not associated with administration of sodium bicarbonate in the treatment of hyperkalemia.
10.	d	Administration of hypertonic glucose solutions will cause potassium to shift into the cells.	a, b, and c. Hyperaldosterone, steroid excess, and potassium-deficient TPN will also cause an electrolyte shift, but not necessarily that described in the stem.

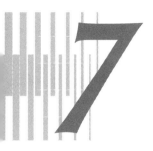

7 Chloride: Normal and Altered Balance

I. Normal balance

A. Description
   1. Chloride is the major anion in extracellular fluid (ECF).
   2. Normal values: Serum chloride levels range from 95 to 108 mEq/L.
B. Supply and sources
   1. Chloride is taken in through the diet, especially from foods rich in salt.
   2. It is found in combination with sodium in the blood as sodium chloride (NaCl).
   3. It is found in combination with hydrogen in the stomach as hydrogen chloride (HCl).
C. Functions
   1. Works with sodium to maintain serum osmolarity.
   2. Maintains the balance of cations in the intracellular fluid (ICF) and ECF.
   3. **Participates in maintaining acid–base balance through a mechanism called the chloride shift:**

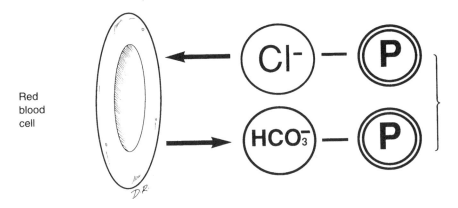

FIGURE 7-1.
The chloride shift. A special carrier protein exchanges chloride and bicarbonate ions into and out of the red blood cells.

    a. Chloride shifts into and out of red blood cells in exchange for bicarbonate to maintain acid–base balance (Fig. 7-1).

    b. As part of maintaining acid–base balance, carbonic acid (H_2CO_3), which is formed in the red blood cells (RBCs), separates into H and HCO_3.

    c. The hydrogen ion attaches to hemoglobin, and the HCO_3 is free to leave the RBCs and circulate in the plasma; if this were to occur, there would be an excess of HCO_3 in the plasma.

    d. However, as HCO_3 diffuses out of the RBCs and into the plasma, chloride shifts into the RBCs to maintain electrical neutrality in the RBCs.

    e. A special protein (known as the bicarbonate-chloride carrier protein) shifts these two electrolytes back and forth into and out of the RBCs.

D. Regulation

    1. Chloride is regulated by renal and extrarenal mechanisms.

    2. *Renal regulation:*

        a. Plasma concentration of chloride is regulated by the kidneys through reabsorption and is equal to the amount of chloride filtered through the glomerulus.

        b. Chloride reabsorption depends on sodium reabsorption, which is regulated by aldosterone in the distal tubule and collecting ducts. Any alteration in sodium reabsorption will secondarily affect the chloride level.

        c. Chloride is excreted in the urine; the amount excreted is related to the amount taken in through the diet or intravenous infusion or to the amount needed by the body.

    3. *Extrarenal regulation:*

        a. Chloride is absorbed in the bowel (mainly the duodenum and jejunum) as it passively follows sodium to maintain electrical neutrality across the bowel wall.

    b.   Chloride also is actively absorbed in the ileum and large intestine by a specialized transport mechanism.

    c.   In this transport mechanism, a number of chloride ions are reabsorbed for an equal number of secreted bicarbonate ions; bicarbonate moves directly from the serum into the bowel and is exchanged for chloride ions to maintain electrical neutrality.

    d.   This mechanism allows bicarbonate to neutralize acids created by intestinal bacteria.

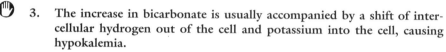

II. Chloride deficiency: Hypochloremia

A. Description

    1.   Hypochloremia is a condition in which the serum chloride level is below 95 mEq/L.

    2.   When chloride concentrations drop below 95 mEq/L, bicarbonate reabsorption increases proportionally, causing metabolic alkalosis.

    3.   **The increase in bicarbonate is usually accompanied by a shift of intercellular hydrogen out of the cell and potassium into the cell, causing hypokalemia.**

B. Etiology

    1.   Excessive losses through the GI system, such as from:

        a.   Vomiting

        b.   Nasogastric suctioning

        c.   Irrigation

    2.   Sodium deficits related to restricted intake or losses through diuretics

    3.   Losses through the urine due to:

        a.   Diuretic therapy (which can alter various electrolyte levels)

        b.   Chloriduria (excessive excretion of chloride in the urine); this condition, which usually results from increased chloride intake, commonly occurs in patients with Bartter's syndrome who are receiving potassium chloride to treat hypokalemia. Another possible cause of chloriduria is a defect of sodium reabsorption in the renal tubules.

    4.   Chloridorrhea, a congenital disorder that presents with frequent loose stools, resulting in increased loss of hydrochloric acid and increased renal hydrogen excretion

    5.   Excessive water within the body (eg, due to overinfusion of hypotonic solutions or excessive water intake); known as dilutional hypochloremia

C. Assessment findings

    1.   No specific symptoms are associated with hypochloremia, which usually occurs secondary to other pathophysiologic processes (eg, cystic fibrosis) along with changes in other electrolytes.

    2.   Laboratory tests reveal serum chloride level below 95 mEq/L.

D. Potential nursing diagnoses

    1.   High Risk for Injury

2. Fluid Volume Excess/Deficit (depending on the cause)

E. Interventions

1. Assist in achieving the treatment objective of restoring the chloride level within the range of 95 to 108 mEq/L.
2. Institute measures to manage the underlying disorder.
3. Replace fluids, as ordered, to restore and maintain serum osmolarity.
4. Replace electrolytes as needed to maintain acid–base balance.
5. Monitor serum electrolytes.

F. Evaluation

1. Serum chloride level returns to a range between 95 and 108 mEq/L.
2. Serum electrolyte levels remain in normal ranges.
3. The underlying disorder is corrected.
4. The patient's fluid volume is normal.
5. The patient is free from injury.

III.   Chloride excess: Hyperchloremia

A. Description: Serum chloride level above 108 mEq/L.

B. Etiology

1. Sodium excess (hypernatremia)
2. Bicarbonate deficit (metabolic acidosis)

C. Assessment findings

1. No specific symptoms are associated with hyperchloremia, which usually occurs secondary to other electrolyte disorders.
2. **Hyperchloremia can occur with hypernatremia or metabolic acidosis.**
3. Laboratory tests reveal serum chloride level above 108 mEq/L.

D. Potential nursing diagnoses vary with coexisting disorder.

1. Fluid Volume Deficit
2. High Risk for Injury

E. Interventions

1. Identify patient at risk, especially those using diuretics.
2. Institute measures to manage the underlying disorder.
3. Monitor serum electrolytes.
4. Monitor fluid intake and output.
5. Monitor urinary concentration of chloride.
6. Monitor the patient's ingestion of chloride from sources such as table salt, fruit, vegetables, and excess water intake.

F. Evaluation

1. Serum chloride level returns to a range between 95 and 108 mEq/L.
2. Serum electrolyte levels remain in normal ranges.
3. The underlying disorder is corrected.
4. The patient's fluid volume is normal.
5. The patient is free of injury.

Bibliography

Bullock, B. (1996). *Pathophysiology: Adaptations and alterations in function* (4th ed.). Philadelphia: J. B. Lippincott.

Drummer, C., Gerzer, R., Heer, M., et al. (1992). Effects of an acute saline infusion on fluid and electrolyte metabolism in humans. *American Journal of Physiology,* May, 744–754.

Guyton, A. (1991). *Textbook of medical physiology* (8th ed.). Philadelphia: W. B. Saunders.

Kinney, M., Packa, D., & Dunbar, S. (1993). *AACN's clinical reference for critical-care nursing* (3rd ed.). St. Louis: C.V. Mosby.

Kokko, J., & Tannen, R. (1996). *Fluids and electrolytes* (3rd ed.). Philadelphia: W. B. Saunders.

Metheny, N. (1996). *Fluid and electrolyte balance: Nursing considerations* (3rd ed.). Philadelphia: J. B. Lippincott.

Miller, M. (1997). Fluid and electrolyte homeostasis in the elderly: physiologic changes of aging and clinical consequences. *Baillieres Clinical Endocrinology and Metabolism,* 11(2), 367–387.

Narrins, R. (Ed). (1994). *Maxwell & Kleemans clinical disorders of fluid and electrolyte metabolism* (5th ed.). New York: McGraw-Hill.

North American Nursing Diagnosis Association. Nursing Diagnosis: Definitions and Classifications. The Auth. 1996.

Plante, G. E., Chakir, M., Lehoux, S., & Lortie, M. (1995). Disorders of body fluid balance: A new look into the mechanisms of disease. *Canadian Journal of Cardiology,* 11(9), 788–802.

Porth, C. (1994). *Pathophysiology: Concepts of altered health states* (4th ed.). Philadelphia: J. B. Lippincott.

Rose, B. (1994). *Clinical physiology of acid-base and electrolyte disorders* (4th ed.). New York: McGraw-Hill.

Seaman, S. L. (1995). Renal physiology part II: Fluid and electrolyte regulation. *Neonatal network,* 14(5), 5–11.

Smith, K., & Brain, E. (1991). *Fluids and electrolytes: A conceptual approach* (2nd ed.). New York: Churchill Livingstone.

Szerlip, H., & Goldfarb, S. (1993). *Workshops in fluid and electrolyte disorders.* New York: Churchill Livingstone.

Toto, K. (1994). Endocrine physiology. *Critical Care Nursing Clinics of North America,* December, 647–657.

STUDY QUESTIONS

1. On admission, a patient's serum chloride level is 90 mEq/L. The nurse interprets this as:
   a. low
   b. high
   c. within the normal range
   d. unable to be interpreted

2. Chloride is a major anion found in the extracellular fluid (ECF); chloride levels fluctuate in response to:
   a. H_2O levels
   b. potassium levels
   c. HCO_3 levels
   d. hemoglobin levels

3. Hypochloremia may be associated with:
   a. starvation
   b. excessive water intake
   c. insulin therapy
   d. decreased water intake

4. When assessing a patient for hyperchloremia, the nurse would expect to find which of the following concurrent conditions?
   a. metabolic alkalosis
   b. hyponatremia
   c. hypernatremia
   d. excessive bicarbonate

5. Chloridorrhea is a congenital disorder typically resulting in:
   a. decreased HCO_3 production
   b. excessive potassium
   c. excessive HCL loss
   d. decreased renal hydrogen excretion

6. When caring for a patient with gastrointestinal disease, the nurse is aware that which of the following therapies might cause chloride loss?
   a. retention enemas
   b. cathartics
   c. nasogastric suctioning
   d. nasogastric tube feeding

7. Hypochloremia is associated with which of the following electrolyte disorders?
   a. hyperkalemia
   b. hyponatremia
   c. hypermagnesemia
   d. hyperphosphatemia

8. Chloride shift exchanges chloride for which of the following electrolytes?
   a. sodium
   b. potassium
   c. bicarbonate
   d. hydrogen

9. The chloride shift occurs in which structure:
   a. red blood cells
   b. white blood cells
   c. platelets
   d. kidney

10. The nurse knows that treatment for hypochloremia is successful when the serum chloride level is:
    a. 3.5–5.0 mEq/L
    b. 100–200 mEq/L
    c. 30–40 mEq/L
    d. 95–108 mEq/L

ANSWER KEY

Question	Correct answer	Correct answer rationale	Incorrect answer rationales
1.	a	Serum chloride level below 95 mEq/L is low, indicating hypochloremia.	b. Serum chloride level above 108 mEq/L is high, indicating hyperchloremia. c. Normal serum chloride levels range from 95 to 108 mEq/L. d. This response is incorrect because laboratory tests can always be interpreted.
2.	c	ECF chloride levels fluctuate with levels of bicarbonate (HCO_3); as HCO_3 levels increase, chloride levels decrease.	a, b, and d. These responses are incorrect because chloride does not shift in response to these situations.
3.	b	Dilutional hypochloremia may be seen in states of excessive water intake.	a, c, and d. Hypochloremia is associated with these situations.
4.	c	Greater than normal amounts of chloride can be expected with hypernatremia.	a. Metabolic acidosis, not alkalosis, is present. b. Hypernatremia, not hyponatremia, is present. d. Decreased, not excessive HCO_3, is present.
5.	c	Chloridorrhea presents with frequent loose stools, resulting in increased loss of HCl.	a, b, and d. Chloridorrhea results in increased HCO_3 production, decreased potassium, and increased renal hydrogen excretion.
6.	c	Nasogastric suctioning may result in excessive chloride loss, since gastric fluid is rich in chlorides.	a, b, and d. These therapies are not related to loss of any electrolytes.
7.	b	Hypochloremia is associated with sodium deficits related to restricted intake or losses through diuretics.	a, c, and d. These electrolyte disorders are not associated with hypochloremia.
8.	c	Chloride exchanges for bicarbonate in the red blood cells, helping to maintain acid–base balance. When the hydrogen ion attaches to hemoglobin, bicarbonate exits and chloride shifts in to maintain electrical neutrality.	a, b, and d. These electrolytes do not exchange for chloride during the chloride shift.
9.	a	The chloride shift occurs in the red blood cell.	c, b, and d. The chloride shift does not occur in these places.
10.	d	Normal serum chloride level is 95–108 mEq/L.	a, b, and c. These are not normal chloride levels.

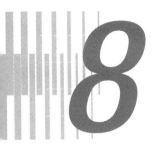

8 Calcium: Normal and Altered Balance

I. Normal balance

A. **Description**
   1. Calcium is a major cation; total body content is about 1200 g.
   2. Normal serum calcium level ranges from 8.5 to 10.5 mg/dL.
   3. Calcium is regulated closely with magnesium and phosphorus.

B. **Supply and sources**

   1. **Most of the total body calcium (99%) is found in bones and teeth.**
   2. **Calcium that is not bound to bone is either bound to plasma protein or is ionized.**
   3. Ionized calcium (calcium that is unattached) performs vital metabolic functions. It is the ionized calcium that is measured in serum chemistry values.
   4. Calcium is taken in through the diet; recommended daily calcium intake is 800 mg.
   5. Abnormal routes of calcium intake include intravenous (IV) administration or hyperalimentation.

C.   Functions

   1.   Calcium is mobilized through a complicated metabolic pathway that involves the endocrine, renal, and gastrointestinal (GI) systems.

2.   Calcium that is bound to bone contributes to bone and tooth rigidity and strength.

3.   Some calcium is bound to protein, so abnormal calcium levels are analyzed in relation to serum protein levels.

4.   Ionized calcium is required as an enzymatic cofactor for many functions, especially blood clotting. Changes in serum calcium will alter blood clotting.

5.   Calcium also is:

   a.   Partially responsible for maintaining cell membrane structure and function

   b.   Required for nerve, muscle, and cardiac conduction by its participation in the sodium-potassium pump

   c.   Required for hormonal secretions

D.   Regulation

1.   *GI regulation:*

   a.   Calcium is absorbed in the GI tract and excreted in the urine.

   b.   Vitamin D in its biologically active form, known as 1,25-dihydroxycholecalciferol (1,25 DHC), is required for the absorption of calcium; this conversion of vitamin D occurs in the kidneys.

2.   *Renal regulation:*

   a.   Calcium is filtered in the glomerulus and reabsorbed in the tubules.

   b.   When excessive calcium is present, it may precipitate to form stones.

3.   *Endocrine regulation:*

   a.   The parathyroid gland responds to low plasma calcium by releasing parathyroid hormone (PTH).

   b.   PTH in turn stimulates the release of calcium from bone into the serum to bring serum levels to normal (Fig. 8-1); over many years, this depletes the bone, contributing to osteoporosis.

   c.   However, if serum phosphorus levels are higher than normal, the calcium will bind with the phosphorus.

   d.   This binding of calcium and phosphorus, known as calcium phosphate or the phosphate product, can be detrimental if the calcium phosphate product exceeds 70 mEq/L. Soft-tissue calcification of the eyes, blood vessels, and cardiac conduction system may occur.

   e.   Calcitonin, a thyroid hormone, moves calcium from plasma to bone when serum levels rise.

II.   Calcium deficiency: Hypocalcemia

A.   Description: Serum calcium level below 8.5 mg/dL

B.   Etiology

1.   Inadequate intake or absorption of calcium due to:

   a.   Anorexia

   b.   Acute or chronic renal failure (in these conditions 1,25 DHC is not produced)

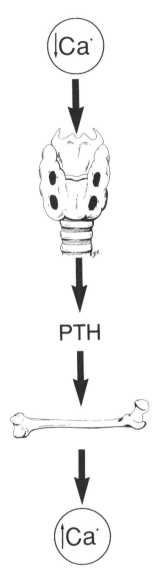

FIGURE 8-1.
PTH and calcium. Decreasing serum calcium levels pull calcium out of bone into serum through the action of PTH.

    c.   Vitamin D deficiency
    d.   Inadequate exposure to ultraviolet light, which hinders conversion of vitamin D to its active form
    e.   Malabsorption of calcium which can result from any GI disease
    f.   Acute pancreatitis which may result in hypocalcemia
    g.   Alcohol abuse which can lead to hypocalcemia as it causes intestinal malabsorption, hypomagnesemia, hypoalbuminemia, and pancreatitis
  2.   Excessive elimination or excretion (eg, as occurs in patients on large doses of Lasix)
  3.   Low PTH levels, which reduce calcium absorption

4. Electrolyte shifts due to:
    a. Hypoparathyroidism, which reduces levels of PTH
    b. Renal failure, which causes hyperphosphatemia; this imbalance reduces serum calcium as the excessive phosphorus binds with ionized calcium. There is always a reciprocal drop in calcium when phosphorous is high because the phosphorous will bind to the calcium, lowering serum values.
    c. Hypomagnesemia which can cause hypocalcemia
5. Alkalosis from any etiology or excessive administration of HCO_3, because the HCO_3 binds with ionized calcium
6. Infusion of citrated blood can lead to transient hypocalcemia because citrate will bind to the ionized calcium and lower serum levels.
7. Some drugs may contribute to or cause hypocalcemia. A partial list is found in Table 8-1.

C. Assessment findings
1. Because calcium is a critical part of neuromuscular contraction, falling calcium levels affect the contraction of smooth, skeletal, and cardiac muscles; symptoms may include:
    a. Muscle cramps in arms and legs
    b. Muscle spasms (spasms in bronchial and laryngeal muscles are particularly dangerous)
    c. Cardiac dysrhythmias (eg, prolonged Q-T interval) (Fig. 8-2)
2. Calcium also is a critical part of nerve cell conduction. Low plasma calcium levels make nerve cells more excitable. This occurs because a lack of calcium causes increased neural permeability to sodium. Manifestations include:
    a. Hyperactive deep-tendon reflexes

TABLE 8-1
Drugs With Calcium-Lowering Effects

DRUG	MECHANISM
Loop diuretics (such as furosemide)	Increases renal excretion of calcium
Anticonvulsants (especially Dilantin and phenobarbital)	Inhibits gastrointestinal calcium absorption and increases vitamin D metabolism
Citrate-buffered blood and blood products	Presumably binds ionized Ca^{2+} with citrate
Phosphates (orally, IV, or enema)	Phosphate combines with calcium
Mithramycin	Decreases calcium mobilization from bone
Calcitonin	Decreases calcium mobilization from bone
Drugs that lower serum Mg level (such as Cisplatin and Gentamycin)	By inducing hypomagnesemia, may decrease calcium mobilization from bone
EDTA (disodium edetate)	Physically combines with calcium for excretion
Alcohol (chronic abuse)	Multiple factors
Certain radiographic contrast media[23]	Those containing chelating agents combine with calcium

(Source: Metheny, N. F&E Balance, 3/e, 1996 Table 6-1, page 119)

    b. Paresthesia of extremities

    c. Positive Chvostek's sign occurs when facial twitching accompanies tapping of the facial nerve.

    d. Trousseau's signs is positive in hypocalcemia. To test for this sign inflate a blood pressure cuff above systolic pressure for about 3 minutes. A carpal spasm will result if the patient is hypocalcemic. Figure 14-1 (page 162) illustrates Trousseau's sign.

    e. Confusion

    f. Moodiness and anxiety

    g. Hypocalcemic tetany and seizures

    h. Electrocardiogram changes usually noted as prolonged Q-T interval (see Fig. 8-2).

3. Because calcium is needed for normal blood clotting, symptoms associated with excessive bleeding may occur; these can include:

    a. Easy bruising and petechiae

    b. Excessive bleeding when cut

4. Laboratory tests reveal:

    a. Serum calcium levels below 8.5 mg/dL

    b. Hyperphosphatemia (because decreased calcium levels result in increased phosphorus levels)

    c. Hypomagnesemia or hypoalbuminemia (because calcium levels are regulated along with magnesium).

    d. albumin (because calcium is bound to it)

    e. Prolonged prothrombin time and partial thromboplastin time (because calcium is required for blood clotting)

D. Potential nursing diagnoses

    1. Ineffective Breathing Patterns related to altered calcium

    2. Decreased Cardiac Output

    3. High Risk for Injury

    4. Pain

    5. Impaired Physical Mobility

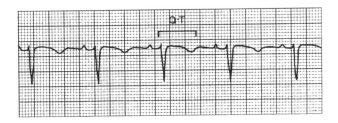

FIGURE 8-2.
Prolonged Q-T interval (hypocalcemia). For this heart rate of 70 beats/min, the Q-T interval should be between 0.31 and 0.38 s. This patient's Q-T interval measures 0.50 s because his serum calcium level is 5.4 mg/dL. (Normal serum calcium is 8.5–10.5 mg/dL).

6. Activity Intolerance
7. Fatigue
8. High Risk for Injury

E. Interventions
1. Identify patients at risk for hypocalcemia (eg, those who have had thyroid disease especially thyroidectomy and those with GI or renal disorders).

 2. **Institute cardiac monitoring, and secure precautions if the patient's calcium level is dangerously low.**
3. Assist in achieving the treatment objective of restoring the calcium level within a range between 8.5 and 10.5 mg/dL.
4. For moderate loss:
   a. Give oral supplements, as ordered, with vitamin D. Be aware that if hyperphosphatemia is present, phosphate supplements also must be given because there is a danger that the calcium supplement will bind with the phosphorus and create an excess calcium phosphate product.
   b. Provide nutritional counseling if hypocalcemia is due to dietary deficiency.
   c. Instruct the patient that exercise enhances calcium mobilization from bone and will replenish plasma calcium levels.
5. For dangerously low levels:
   a. Replace calcium with IV calcium gluconate as ordered. Be aware that a large vein is needed for IV calcium replacement and that infiltration can cause sloughing.
   b. Institute cardiac monitoring.
   c. Administer calcium *with caution* to patients on digoxin, because calcium sensitizes the heart to digoxin.

F. Evaluation
1. Serum calcium level returns to a range between 8.5 and 10.5 mg/dL.
2. The patient's breathing patterns are normal.
3. The patient experiences no bleeding.
4. The patient's cardiac output is normal.
5. The patient is free from injury.

III.   Calcium excess: Hypercalcemia

A. Description: serum calcium level above 10.5 mg/dL
B. Etiology
1. Excessive calcium intake or absorption, such as from:
   a. Overzealous use of calcium supplements
   b. Increased vitamin D intake
   c. Altered GI metabolism
   d. Medications which may contain calcium (eg, calcium-containing antacids and phosphate-binding gels) or elevate calcium. A partial list of calcium-containing over-the-counter products is found in Table 8-2. A partial list of medications that elevate calcium is found in Table 8-3.

 2. **Metabolic conditions, such as:**

TABLE 8-2
Selected Calcium-containing Products for Oral Use

PRODUCT	ELEMENTAL CA CONTENT* (MG/TABLET)	ANION	VITAMIN D CONTENT (IU/TABLET)
Alka 2	200	Carbonate	
Alka-Mints	340	Carbonate	
Biocal	250, 500	Carbonate	
Calcet	153	Carbonate, gluconate, lactate	100
Calcium acetate	167/668 mg	Acetate	
Calcium gluconate	45/500 mg	Gluconate	
Calcium lactate	42/325 mg	Lactate	
Calsup	300, 600	Carbonate	±200
Ca Plus	280	Protein complex	
Calciday	667	Carbonate	
Caltrate	600	Carbonate	±125
Citracal	200 mg/950 mg 500 mg/effervescent tablet	Citrate	
Dical-D	350	Phosphate	400
Neocalglucon	115 (per 5 ml)	Glubionate	
Os Cal	250, 500	Carbonate	
Oystercal	250, 375, 500	Carbonate	
Posture	300, 600	Tricalcium, phosphate	
Titralac	200 400 (per 5 ml)	Carbonate	
Tums	200	Carbonate	

Apers, D. H., Stenson, W. F., Bier, D. M. (1995). Manual of nutritional therapeutics (3rd ed.) © David H. Alpers, William F. Stenson and Dennis M. Bier.
*The contents of anhydrous calcium salts as elemental calcium are as follows: glubionate 6.5%, gluconate 9%, lactate 13%, citrate 21%, acetate 25%, dibasic phosphate 23%, tricalcium phosphate 39%, and carbonate 40%.

      a. **Hyperparathyroidism,** which accelerates PTH effects on bone and removes bound calcium to the serum
      b. **Renal tubule disorders,** which reduce the efficiency of renal electrolyte regulation
      c. **Hypophosphatemia** (because phosphorus and calcium have an inversely reciprocal relationship)
      d. **Thyrotoxicosis,** which accelerates calcitonin secretion
      e. **Bone disorders** (eg, cancers and metastatic lesions, accelerated bone metabolism)
      f. **Immobility,** which alters bone metabolism
   C. **Assessment findings**
      1. Symptom severity increases as the calcium level rises.

TABLE 8-3
Drugs with Calcium-Elevating Effects

DRUG	MECHANISM
Thiazide diuretics	Decrease renal calcium excretion
Lithium	Decreases renal calcium excretion
Prolonged megadoses of vitamins A and D	Vitamin A likely increases calcium mobilization from bone; vitamin D increases GI calcium absorption and mobilization of calcium from bone
Theophylline	Perhaps increases effect of endogenous parathyroid hormone
Milk with soluble alkali (especially calcium carbonate)	Multiple mechanisms

Metheny, N. M. (1996). Fluid and electrolyte balance (3rd ed.). Philadelphia: Lippincott-Raven.

2. **Rising calcium level affects the skeletal, smooth, and cardiac muscles; manifestations may include:**
    a. **Decreased peristalsis, resulting in constipation**
    b. **Muscle weakness or flaccidity**
    c. **Cardiac dysrhythmias, reflected in shortened Q-T interval (Fig. 8-3)**
3. Neurologic manifestations occur because calcium affects conduction across nerve cells; symptoms may include:
    a. Confusion
    b. Personality changes
    c. Altered level of consciousness
    d. Coma
4. Because calcium plays a role in many metabolic processes, manifestations may occur in other systems; these include:
    a. Urinary calculi (may be present as calcium precipitates in the kidney)
    b. GI alterations (eg, anorexia, thirst, nausea, and vomiting)
    c. Pathologic fractures (can result when calcium leaves the bone)
    d. Soft-tissue calcification (can result when calcium levels rise, and the calcium binds to phosphorous. This is known as calcium phosphate and causes calcification)
5. Laboratory and diagnostic tests reveal:
    a. Serum calcium level above 10.5 mg/dL
    b. Bone changes and reduced bone density

D. Potential nursing diagnoses
1. Decreased Cardiac Output
2. High Risk for Injury
3. Constipation
4. Altered Nutrition: Less Than Body Requirements
5. Impaired Memory

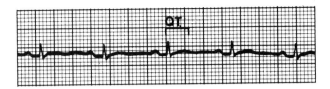

FIGURE 8-3.
Shortened Q-T interval (hypercalcemia). The normal Q-T interval for the above heart rate of 88 beats/min is 0.28 s to 0.36 s. This patient's serum calcium level is 12.1 mg/dL, and the Q-T interval measures 0.24 s.

E.   Interventions

1.   Institute measures to prevent hypercalcemia:
   a.   Recognize high-risk patients, and instruct them to avoid calcium-rich foods.
   b.   Ambulate patients as early as possible.
2.   Institute measures to eliminate excess calcium:
   a.   Administer loop diuretics (e.g., Lasix) as ordered to facilitate calcium removal.
   b.   Administer IV normal saline as ordered to foster diuresis and subsequent calcium elimination.
3.   Administer calcitonin as ordered to lower serum calcium levels.
4.   Monitor electrolyte status.

F.   Evaluation

1.   Serum calcium level returns to normal range.
2.   The patient's cardiac output is normal.
3.   The patient is free from injury.

STUDY QUESTIONS

1. Normal serum calcium levels are:
   a. 800 mg
   b. 1200 mg
   c. 8.5 to 10.5 mg/dl
   d. 2.5 to 4.5 mg/dl

2. Serum calcium levels rise with metastatic bone lesions because of:
   a. hyperphosphatemia
   b. osteoporosis
   c. chemotherapy
   d. accelerated bone metabolism

3. When assessing a patient for hypocalcemia, the nurse would expect to find:
   a. hypoactive deep tendon reflexes
   b. prolonged Q-T interval on EKG
   c. increased muscle strength
   d. decreased peristalsis

4. When educating a patient about foods high in calcium, the nurse would recommend:
   a. canned fish
   b. coffee
   c. dry beans
   d. meat

5. Nursing interventions for a patient with hypocalcemia may include:
   a. encouraging bedrest
   b. administering IV calcium gluconate
   c. administering calcitonin
   d. using loop diuretics

6. When caring for a patient with hypercalcemia, the nurse should plan to administer which of the following drugs?
   a. Inderal
   b. bicarbonate
   c. Lasix
   d. mannitol

7. The most dangerous sequela of hypercalcemia is:
   a. constipation
   b. muscle weakness
   c. dyspnea
   d. dysrhythmias

8. Which one of the following metabolic conditions places a patient at high risk for hypercalcemia?
   a. myxedema
   b. exercise
   c. hyperphosphatemia
   d. hyperparathyroidism

9. Which patient is at the highest risk for hypocalcemia:
   a. Two hours post thyroidectomy
   b. Renal tubular acidosis
   c. Bone disease
   d. Administration of Lasix

10. When a patient is found to have a calcium imbalance the nurse must be sure to assess serum levels of:
    a. Phosphorous
    b. Albumin
    c. Magnesium
    d. All of the above

ANSWER KEY

Question	Correct answer	Correct answer rationale	Incorrect answer rationales
1.	c	Normal calcium level ranges from 8.5 to 10.5 mg/dl.	a, b, and d. These are not the normal levels.
2.	d	Bone cancers and metastatic lesions result in hypercalcemia because of accelerated bone metabolism, which causes calcium to be released from the bone to the blood.	a. Hyperphosphatemia would result in hypocalcemia. b and c. These are not reasons for hypercalcemia that results from bone lesions.
3.	b	Hypocalcemia is reflected as a prolonged Q-T interval on the EKG.	a, c, and d. Hypoactive deep tendon reflexes and increased muscle strength are not signs of hypocalcemia. Decreased peristalsis resulting in constipation is found in patients with hypercalcemia.
4.	a	Canned fish is high in calcium.	b. Coffee is high in potassium. c and d. Dry beans and meat are high in phosphorous.
5.	b	IV calcium gluconate is used for replacement in severe cases of hypocalcemia.	a. Exercise, not bedrest would be recommended to release calcium from the bone into the serum. c and d. Calcitonin and loop diuretics are used to lower serum calcium levels.
6.	c	Lasix is a loop diuretic; this type of diuretic facilitates calcium removal.	a and b. These drugs will not facilitate calcium removal. d. Mannitol is an osmotic diuretic, and treatment of hypercalcemia requires administration of a loop diuretic.
7.	d	Hypercalcemia causes cardiac dysrhythmias, reflected in a shortened Q-T interval.	a and b. Constipation and muscle weakness are sequelae of hypercalcemia, but are not dangerous. c. Dyspnea is not a sequela of hypercalcemia.
8.	d	Hyperparathyroidism accelerates parathyroid hormone (PTH) effects on bone and removes bound calcium into the serum.	a. Myxedema is associated with hypothyroidism. Hyperthyroidism, or thyrotoxicosis, is the direct opposite of hypothyroidism; it is thyrotoxicosis that places a patient at risk. b. Exercise places a patient at less risk; immobility causes hypercalcemia. c. Hypophosphatemia is associated with hypercalcemia.

Question	Correct answer	Correct answer rationale	Incorrect answer rationales
9.	a	A patient who has had recent thyroidectomy may have had inadvertent removal of the parathyroid gland, which is responsible for calcium regulation.	b and c. Patients with renal tubular acidosis and bone disease are at risk for hypercalcemia. d. Lasix will eliminate calcium, but patient in *a* is at a higher risk.
10.	d	All of these levels must be evaluated because their regulation is interconnected.	

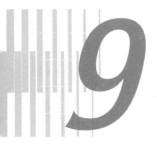

9 Magnesium: Normal and Altered Balance

I. Normal balance

A. Description

    1. Magnesium is the second most abundant cation in the intracellular fluid.

    2. Normal serum magnesium concentration ranges from 1.3 to 2.1 mEq/L.

B. Supply and sources

    1. Magnesium is taken in through the diet and eliminated through the kidneys and gastrointestinal system.

    2. Abnormal routes of magnesium intake include:

        a. IV administration

        b. Hyperalimentation

    3. Only 1% of total body magnesium is ionized.

    4. The remaining magnesium is bound to bone (above 60%) or contained inside the cells.

C. Functions

    1. Exerts its effect on the myoneural junction, affecting neuromuscular irritability

    2. Assists in contraction of cardiac and skeletal muscle cells

    3. Contributes to vasodilation and through this effect, changes blood pressure and cardiac output

    4. Activates intracellular enzymes to participate in carbohydrate and protein metabolism

    5. Facilitates sodium and potassium transport across the cell membrane

    6. Influences intracellular calcium levels through its effect on parathyroid hormone secretion

D. **Regulation**

    1. Magnesium regulation is not clearly understood, but factors that influence the balance of other cations affect magnesium as well.

    2. **As the second most abundant intracellular cation, its renal regulation parallels potassium.**

        a. Magnesium is filtered along with all other electrolytes in the glomerulus.

        b. The amount filtered depends on the amount present.

        c. Magnesium is reabsorbed across all segments of the renal tubules.

        d. Tubular reabsorption is affected by the presence of the magnesium ion, especially in Henle's loop.

        e. When extracellular magnesium is high, excess magnesium is excreted.

        f. When extracellular magnesium is low, magnesium is conserved.

        g. Tubules can conserve magnesium so that daily losses can be reduced to 1.0 mEq/L per day.

        h. Diuretics that act on this region (eg, Lasix) can greatly increase magnesium excretion.

    3. Extrarenal regulation

        a. Dietary magnesium is absorbed in the jejunum and ileum.

        b. When a deficiency exists, absorption is increased.

        c. Parathyroid and steroid hormones play a role in magnesium regulation.

II. Magnesium deficiency: Hypomagnesemia

A. **Description: Serum magnesium levels less than 1.3 mEq/L**

B. **Etiology**

    1. Magnesium loss, such as from:

        a. Severe GI fluid losses due to vomiting, diarrhea, gastric suctioning, or diuretics

        b. Fluids lost from the bowel (These fluids have a high magnesium content when compared to the stomach so losses from the lower GI tract cause hypomagnesemia faster than upper GI losses).

        c. Burns and debridement therapy

        d. Administration of loop diuretics

    2. Inadequate intake or absorption due to:

        a. Malnutrition or starvation

        b. Malabsorption syndrome

      c.   Excessive dietary intake of calcium or vitamin D

  3. Alcohol intake may cause hypomagnesia because of increased GI losses and malabsorption.

  4. Fluid and electrolyte shifts due to:

      a.   Administration of hyperalimentation solutions that are magnesium deficient

      b.   Hypercalcemia

      c.   Hypoparathyroidism

      d.   Hypoaldosteronism (in which sodium is not absorbed and therefore magnesium is not absorbed)

      e.   High-dose steroid use

      f.   Diabetic ketoacidosis

      g.   Sepsis

      h.   Pancreatitis

      i.   Alcoholism

      j.   Pregnancy-induced hypertension

      k.   Refeeding after starvation

  5. Renal disease may cause hypomagnesemia (as well as hypermagnesemia, depending on the disease).

  6. Administration of certain medications, such as Gentamicin or, cancer chemotherapy (especially Cisplatin).

C. **Assessment findings**

  1. Clinical manifestations may include vomiting or diarrhea; however, these symptoms may be the cause of hypomagnesemia.

  2. Because magnesium is required for neuromuscular and cardiac muscle contraction and for vasodilation, any alteration will affect those muscle systems.

  3. Cardiovascular symptoms include:

      a.   Dysrhythmia

      b.   Hypotension

      c.   Increased possibility of digoxin toxicity

  4. **Symptoms of hypomagnesemia are more severe in the neuromuscular system and include:**

      a.   **Tetany**

      b.   **Seizures**

      c.   **Confusion**

      d.   **Tremors**

      e.   **Hyperactive deep-tendon reflexes**

      f.   **Laryngeal stridor**

      g.   **Positive Chvostek's and Trousseau's signs**

      h.   **Memory loss**

  3. Laboratory results reveal:

      a.   Serum magnesium level below 1.3 mEq/L

      b.   Hypocalcemia

      c.   Hypokalemia

  4. Another diagnostic cue is electrocardiogram (EKG) changes, which reveal prolonged PR and T intervals, wide ME complexes, depressed ST segment, and inverted T waves.

D. **Potential nursing diagnoses**
1. High Risk for Injury
2. Decreased Cardiac Output
3. Altered Nutrition: Less Than Body Requirements
4. Potential for Fluid Volume Deficit
5. Impaired Memory

E. **Interventions**

1. **Prevent hypomagnesemia or ensure early detection by identifying high-risk patients (eg, those with anorexia, nausea, vomiting, and diarrhea) and providing appropriate patient education.**
2. Aid in achieving treatment objective of elevating the magnesium level within the range of 1.5 to 2.5 mEq/L.
3. Monitor patients with hypokalemia for impending hypomagnesemia.
4. Monitor patients receiving total parenteral nutrition without magnesium added.
5. Monitor a patient with hypomagnesemia who is on digoxin for signs of digitalis toxicity.
6. Monitor cardiac status.
7. Institute seizure precautions.

8. **Administer magnesium replacement with *extreme* caution and slowly as ordered; rapid administration can cause cardiac arrest. Display 9-1 describes details the nurse must be aware of in administering magnesium replacement.**
9. Monitor urine output, which must be at least 100 mL every 4 hours for adequate renal excretion of magnesium to occur.
10. Assess deep-tendon reflexes; if reflexes are absent, hold the dose, and notify the doctor.
11. Infuse 10% magnesium at rate no more than 1.5 mL/min.
12. Monitor potassium levels closely.
13. Assess for stridor, because hypomagnesemia may cause airway obstruction.
14. Assess for dysphagia.
15. Monitor vital signs and cardiac rhythms.
16. Instruct the patient on diuretics about the dangers of hypomagnesemia.
17. Teach the patient about foods high in magnesium (eg, green vegetables, nuts, and fruit).

F. **Evaluation**
1. Serum magnesium level returns to a range between 1.3 and 2.1 mEq/L.
2. The patient remains free from injury.
3. The patient's cardiac output is normal.

III.   Magnesium excess: Hypermagnesemia

A. **Description: Serum magnesium level above 2.1 mEq/L**
B. **Etiology**
1. Magnesium gain, such as from:
   a. Medications (eg, antacids)
   b. Hyperalimentation administration

DISPLAY 9-1
Nursing Considerations in Administering IV Magnesium

1. The extent of magnesium replacement needed for specific hypomagnesemic patients may vary widely according to (a) the severity of the magnesium deficiency, and (b) the current level of renal function. Generally, the more severe the symptoms, the more aggressive the therapy must be.

2. Carefully check the order for IV magnesium. Be sure that it stipulates one of the following:
   A. Concentration of the solution to be administered (as well as the number of milliliters), fluid in which it is to be diluted, and the time frame over which it is to be given. For example: "Give 2 mL of 50% $MgSO_4$, diluted in 100 mL of 0.9% sodium chloride, over one hr."
   B. Number of grams of magnesium sulfate to be administered, along with the required dilution, and time frame over which it is to be administered. For example: "Give 1 g of $MgSO_4$, diluted in 100 mL of 0.9% sodium chloride, over one hr."
   Recall that magnesium sulfate ($MgSO_4$) is available in concentrations of 10%, 20%, and 50%. One gram of magnesium sulfate is contained in 10 mL of a 10% solution, 5 mL of a 20% solution, and 2 mL of a 50% solution. Obviously, serious errors can occur if the wrong concentration is used.

3. Never accept order for "amps" or "vials" without further specifications.

4. Use IV magnesium with great caution in patients with impaired renal function (as evidenced by an elevated serum creatinine level). Recall that the primary route of magnesium excretion is via the kidneys; thus, it is easy to induce hypermagnesemia when renal impairment is present. If magnesium replacement is required in a patient with renal impairment, the physician will probably reduce the dose to be administered by 25% to 50% of that needed for a patient with normal renal function.

5. Monitor urine output at regular intervals throughout the magnesium infusion. It should be maintained at a level of at least 100 mL every 4 hr. An output less than this amount raises the question of adequate urinary elimination of magnesium.

6. Check deep tendon reflexes (such as patellar "knee jerk") before each dose of magnesium, or periodically during continuous infusion of the drug. If reflexes are absent, do not give additional magnesium, and notify the physician. (Because deep tendon reflexes are decreased before adverse respiratory and cardiac effects occur, the presence of knee jerks can usually be relied on to indicate that life-threatening hypermagnesemia is not present.)

7. Therapeutic doses of magnesium can produce flushing and sweating because magnesium acts peripherally to produce vasodilation. Inform the patient that this might occur to minimize concern.

8. Check blood pressure, pulse, and respirations every 15 minutes and monitor the serum magnesium level at regular intervals. Look for a sharp fall in blood pressure or respiratory distress; both are signs of hypermagnesemia. (This can be induced rather easily with improper doses of magnesium.) Patients receiving very aggressive magnesium therapy should receive close cardiac monitoring.

9. If the patient displays signs of severe hypermagnesemia, stop IV administratoion of magnesium and run in the IV solution from the primary line (as appropriate) to keep the vein open. Nofity the physician and be prepared to administer artificial ventilation and IV calcium (if prescribed).

10. Because magnesium is primarily an intracellular ion, it may take several days to completely correct cellular deficits. Therefore, normal serum magnesium values do not necessarily imply that the magnesium depletion has been corrected.

(Source: Metheny, N. M. (1996). Fluid and electrolyte balance (3rd ed.). Philadelphia: Lippincott-Raven.)

    c.   Hemodialysis using hard water dialysate
  2.   Inadequate excretion due to:
    a.   Reduced renal output
    b.   Renal failure
  3.   Fluid and electrolyte shifts due to:

        a.   Hypoadrenalism (by the same mechanism affecting potassium)

        b.   Diabetic ketoacidosis (as glucose brings cations across the cell)

C.   **Assessment findings**

    1.   Because magnesium is responsible for neuromuscular transmission, symptoms of hypermagnesemia are similar to those of hyperkalemia. Clinical manifestations may include:

        a.   Cardiac arrhythmias

        b.   Vasodilation (which causes hypotension, flushing, and warm systemic sensations)

        c.   Bradycardia

        d.   Hypoactive deep-tendon reflexes

        e.   Depressed respirations

        f.   Depressed neuromuscular activity

    2.   Laboratory tests reveal serum magnesium level above 2.1 mEq/L.

    3.   EKG reveals changes in PR interval, ME complex, and Q-T.

D.   **Potential nursing diagnoses**

    1.   Decreased Cardiac Output

    2.   Ineffective Breathing Pattern

E.   **Interventions**

    1.   Prevent hypermagnesemia or ensure early detection by identifying high-risk patients (eg, those taking antacids for any reason or receiving hyperalimentation) and providing appropriate patient education.

    2.   Administer calcium gluconate as ordered to antagonize the cardiac effects of magnesium and temporarily relieve symptoms.

    3.   Assess neuromuscular system for deficits.

    4.   Monitor vital signs and cardiac rhythm.

    5.   Check medications for magnesium, especially in patients with renal disorders.

F.   **Evaluation**

    1.   Serum magnesium level returns to normal range.

    2.   The patient's cardiac output is normal.

    3.   The patient's breathing patterns are normal.

Bibliography

Bullock, B. (1996). *Pathophysiology: Adaptions and alterations in function* (4th ed.). Philadelphia: Lippincott.

Davidson, J. K. (1991). *Clinical diabetes mellitus: A problem oriented approach* (2nd ed.). New York: Theime.

Ganong, W. F. (1997). *Review of medical physiology* (18th ed.). Connecticut: Appleton and Lange.

Greenspan, F., & Strewler G. (Eds). (1997) *Basic and clinical endocrinology* (5th ed.). Connecticut: Appleton & Lange.

Guyton, A. C., and Hall, J. E. (1996). *Textbook of medical physiology* (9th ed.). Philadelphia: Saunders.

Ignatavicius, D., & Bayne, M. (1991). *Medical-surgical. A nursing process approach.* Philadelphia: W. B. Saunders.

Kinney, M., Packa, D., & Dunbar, S. (1993). *AACN's clinical reference for critical-care nursing* (3rd ed.). St. Louis: C. V. Mosby.

McCance, K. L., & Huether, S. E. (1994). *Pathophysiology: The biologic basis for disease in adults and children* (2nd ed.). St. Louis: Mosby–Year Book.

Peragallo-Dittko, V. (1993). *Core curriculum for diabetes education* (2nd ed.). Chicago: American Association of Diabetes Educators.

Porth, C. (1994). *Pathophysiology: Concepts of altered health states* (4th ed.). Philadelphia: Lippincott-Raven.

Thelan, L., Davie, J., et al. (1994). *Critical care nursing diagnosis and management* (2nd ed.). St. Louis: C. V. Mosby.

Wilson, J. D. & Foster, D. W. (Eds). (1997) *Williams textbook of endocrinology* (9th ed.). Philadelphia: Saunders.

STUDY QUESTIONS

1. Normal serum magnesium concentrations range from:
   a. 0.5 to 1.5 mEq/L
   b. 1.3 to 2.1 mEq/L
   c. 10.0 to 12.0 mEq/L
   d. 3.5 to 5.0 mEq/L

2. When assessing a patient for hypomagnesemia, the nurse would *not* expect to find:
   a. hyperactive deep tendon reflexes
   b. hypertension
   c. cardiac dysrhythmia
   d. diaphoresis

3. Which of the following groups of patients would the nurse closely monitor as being at high risk for hypomagnesemia?
   a. constipated patients
   b. anorexic patients
   c. obese patients
   d. patients with vitamin D deficiency

4. Nursing interventions for a patient with hypomagnesemia include:
   a. rapidly infusing 10% magnesium IV
   b. increasing diuretic therapy
   c. observing for signs of digitalis toxicity
   d. administering calcium gluconate

5. Which of the following foods selected by a patient with hypermagnesemia indicate the need for additional education?
   a. green vegetables, nuts, and fruit
   b. milk and cheese
   c. orange juice and bananas
   d. bacon and eggs

6. Which of the following findings would the nurse expect to assess in a patient with hypermagnesemia?
   a. serum level 1.2 mEq/L
   b. tachycardia
   c. warm systemic sensation
   d. hypertension

7. When assessing a patient for hypermagnesemia, the nurse is aware that a patient with which of the following conditions is at low risk?
   a. diabetic ketoacidosis
   b. chronic heartburn
   c. hypokalemia
   d. hypoadrenalism

8. Nursing interventions for a patient with hypermagnesemia include:
   a. administering 10% magnesium
   b. withholding diuretics
   c. limiting antacids
   d. administering digitalis

9. A nurse should suspect hypomagnesemia in a patient with:
   a. renal failure on dialysis
   b. respiratory disease with alcoholism
   c. diabetic ketoacidosis on insulin
   d. sudden paralysis who is on Cisplatin

10. When administering replacement magnesium intravenously, the nurse should:
   a. administer the drug with calcium
   b. provide water to prevent dehydration
   c. give the drug very slowly
   d. administer the drug as fast as possible

ANSWER KEY

Question	Correct answer	Correct answer rationale	Incorrect answer rationales
1.	b	Normal serum magnesium concentration ranges from 1.3 to 2.1 mEq/L.	a, c, and d. These are not normal magnesium levels.
2.	c	Cardiac dysrhythmia may be a sign of hypomagnesemia.	a, b, and d. Hypoactive deep tendon reflexes, hypertension, and diaphoresis are not associated with hypomagnesemia.
3.	b	Patients at high risk for hypomagnesemia include anorexics, and those with nausea, vomiting, and diarrhea.	a, c, and d. Vitamin deficiency, obesity, and constipation do not increase the risk of magnesium imbalance.
4.	c	It is important to observe a patient with hypomagnesemia who is taking digitalis for signs of digitalis toxicity.	a. The nurse should infuse 10% magnesium slowly. b. Increasing diuretic therapy can produce hypokalemia, which would would worsen hypomagnesemia. d. Calcium gluconate is given in hypermagnesemia.
5.	a	Green vegetables, nuts, and fruits are good dietary sources of magnesium and would be contraindicated for a patient with hypermagnesemia.	b, c, and d. These responses are incorrect.
6.	c	A warm systemic sensation is a common symptom of hypermagnesemia.	a. Serum magnesium level of 1.2 mEq/L indicates hypomagnesemia. b. Bradycardia, not tachycardia is observed in hypermagnesemia. d. Hypotension, not hypertension occurs in hypermagnesemia.
7.	c	Patients with hyperkalemia, not hypokalemia, are at increased risk to develop hypermagnesemia.	a, b, and d. Diabetic ketoacidosis, increased ingestion of antacids (due to chronic heartburn), and hypoadrenalism also increase a patient's risk for hypermagnesemia.
8.	c	Limiting antacids, which are high in magnesium, is indicated for the patient with hypermagnesemia.	a. 10% magnesium infusion is used to treat hypomagnesemia. b. Withholding diuretics would not help, since diuretics may be part of the treatment. d. Digitalis is not part of the treatment for hypermagnesemia.

Question	Correct answer	Correct answer rationale	Incorrect answer rationales
9.	d	This patient poses the highest risk. Cisplatin is known to deplete the body of magnesium, and sudden paralysis indicated that the nervous system is effected—a hallmark sign of hypomagnesemia.	a and c. These patients are at risk for hypermagnesemia. b. Alcoholism is a risk factor for hypomagnesemia, but letter d is the best answer because the patient already has symptoms.
10.	c	All intravenous drugs must be given slowly. Magnesium must be given slowly because it causes rapid vasodilation, hypotension, and cardiac arrhythmias.	a, b, and c. These are not interventions for intravenous administration of magnesium.

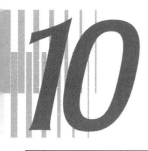

Phosphorus: Normal and Altered Balance

I. Normal balance

A. Description

1. Phosphorus is the major anion in the intracellular fluid (ICF); its concentration inside cells is approximately 100 mEq/L.
2. Normal serum phosphorus concentration ranges from 2.5 to 4.5 mg/dL.

B. Supply and sources

1. Normal sources of phosphorus intake include almost all foods; dairy products are especially rich in phosphorus.
2. Abnormal sources of potassium intake include intravenous administration and hyperalimentation.
3. Eighty percent of phosphorus exists in bone, where it is combined with calcium.
4. The remaining 20% is found in the ICF and extracellular fluid.

C. Functions

1. Acts as the critical component of the phosphate buffer system to aid renal regulation of acids and bases

2.   **Is necessary for the creation of energy (ATP) through cellular metabolism, in which enzymatic action splits the compound adenosine triphosphate to produce phosphate and energy**

3.   Is an essential component of bones and teeth

4.   Maintains cell membrane integrity by binding with lipids to create the phospholipid cell membrane layer

5.   Is critical for the metabolism of protein, carbohydrates, and fats

6.   Is essential to the function of red blood cells, muscles, and the neurologic system

7.   Is a component of DNA and RNA

D.   **Regulation**

1.   Phosphorus is filtered by the glomerulus.

    2.   **When glomerular filtration increases, phosphorus reabsorption decreases; when glomerular filtration decreases, phosphorus reabsorption increases.**

3.   Phosphorus is reabsorbed in the proximal tubule along with sodium.

4.   When parathyroid hormone (PTH) is present, tubular reabsorption is inhibited, increasing phosphorus excretion.

5.   PTH is secreted in response to lowered serum calcium levels and is inhibited with higher serum calcium levels. This PTH secretion in response to calcium helps regulate phosphorus, because phosphorus is found in proportions inversely reciprocal to calcium.

II.   **Phosphorus deficiency: Hypophosphatemia**

A.   Description: Serum phosphorus level below 2.5 mg/dL

B.   Etiology

1.   Inadequate intake or absorption, such as that due to anorexia or malabsorption syndrome

2.   Excessive losses from the gastrointestinal or genitourinary tract, such as from vomiting or diuretic use

3.   Electrolyte shifts in which cations are exchanged (eg, hypokalemia, hypomagnesemia, metabolic acidosis, respiratory alkalosis, hyperaldosteronism)

4.   Administration of high glucose solutions without phosphorus. Higher levels of glucose cause an increase in insulin secretion, which fosters intracellular transport of glucose and phosphorous.

5.   Secondary to diseases such as alcoholism or acute gout

6.   Endocrine disorders, such as:
a.   hyperparathyroidism,
b.   diabetic ketoacidosis which causes urinary phosphate loss when glycosuria, ketonuria, and polyuria are present. Administration of insulin causes the same type of intracellular shift as described above.

7.   Excessive losses through the skin which may result from burns.

    8.   **Nutritional recovery syndrome, also known as "refeeding" syndrome as carbohydrates are introduced. During anabolism there is a rapid intracellular influx of phosphorous.**

9. Use of phosphate binding medications (Amphojel, Basalgel) (especially if there is more drug present than taken in the diet).

C. **Assessment findings**

    1. Neurologic symptoms of ATP deficiency include:
        a. Confusion
        b. Fatigue
        c. Muscle weakness/numbness/paresthesia
        d. Seizures/coma
        e. Nystagmus

    2. Hematologic symptoms include:
        a. Hemolytic anemia (red blood cells are deficient in 2,3-DPG from low phosphorous)
        b. Reduction in oxygen transport results in fatigue and other anemic symptoms.
        c. Platelet dysfunction

    3. Muscle weakness from reduction in ATP
    4. Respiratory weakness from respiratory muscle fatigue
    5. Laboratory tests reveal:
        a. Serum phosphorus levels below 2.5 mg/dL
        b. Hypercalcemia
        c. Rising creatinine phosphokinase levels (if serum phosphorus level remains low)

D. **Potential nursing diagnoses**

    1. Ineffective Breathing Pattern
    2. Fatigue
    3. High Risk for Injury
    4. Impaired Mobility

E. **Interventions**

    1. Prevent hypophosphatemia, and ensure early detection by identifying high-risk patients (eg, those receiving excessive phosphate-binding medications, such as aluminum hydroxide [Amphojel] and aluminum carbonate [Basaljel], or those with hypercalcemia) and providing appropriate patient education.
    2. Assist in the treatment objective of returning the serum phosphorus level to a range between 2.5 to 4.5 mg/dL.
    3. Assess for signs of hypercalcemia, which occurs in the presence of hypophosphatemia.
    4. Increase dietary intake of phosphorus.
    5. Administer parenteral phosphorus as ordered if the depletion is severe.

F. **Evaluation**

    1. Serum phosphorus level returns to a range between 2.5 and 4.5 mg/dL.
    2. The patient remains free of injury.
    3. The patient's breathing pattern is normal.

III. **Phosphorus excess: Hyperphosphatemia**

A. Description: Serum phosphorus level above 4.5 mg/dL
B. Etiology

1. Increased intestinal absorption due to excessive intake of vitamin D
2. Ingestion of excessive quantities of milk or other dairy products high in phosphorous.
3. Ingestion of certain phosphorus-containing medications (eg, laxatives)
4. Administration of phosphorus-containing enemas (eg, Fleet's Phospho-soda)
5. Renal insufficiency or failure where hypocalcemia is present and dietary phosphorous not excreted.
6. Cellular destruction (eg, cancer chemotherapy, trauma, rhabdomyolysis), which causes release of phosphates into the serum
7. Hypoparathyroidism, in which decreased PTH levels reduce calcium concentration, which in turn causes hyperphosphatemia
8. Conditions that result in osteoporosis, because phosphorus is removed from bone and enters the serum

C. **Assessment findings**
1. Manifestations may include:
   a. Muscle spasms, pain, or weakness
   b. Positive Chvostek's or Trousseau's signs
2. Long-term effects are seen in the form of soft-tissue calcification (eg, joints, blood vessels, cornea), usually in patients with renal failure.
3. Laboratory tests show serum phosphorus level above 4.5 mg/dL and the presence of hypocalcemia.

D. **Potential nursing diagnoses**
1. Pain
2. Decreased Cardiac Output
3. Impaired Mobility
4. High Risk for Injury

E. **Interventions**
1. Prevent hyperphosphatemia, and ensure early detection by identifying high-risk patients (eg, those with hypocalcemia) and providing appropriate patient education.
2. Assist in the treatment objective of reducing serum phosphorus levels to a range between 2.5 and 4.5 mg/dL.
3. Administer phosphate-binding medications (eg, aluminum hydroxide) as ordered.
4. Administer calcium supplements along with phosphate binders as ordered for a patient with renal-related hyperphosphatemia.
5. Prepare the patient for hemodialysis, which may remove excessive phosphorus.
6. Instruct the patient to avoid foods and medications containing phosphorus.

F. **Evaluation**
1. Serum phosphorus level returns to a range between 2.5 and 4.5 mg/dL
2. The patient's cardiac output is normal.
3. The patient is free of pain.

Bibliography

Bullock, B. (1996). *Pathophysiology: Adaptions and alterations in function* (4th ed.). Philadelphia: Lippincott.

Davidson, J. K. (1991). *Clinical diabetes mellitus: A problem oriented approach* (2nd ed.). New York: Theime.

Ganong, W. F. (1997). *Review of medical physiology* (18th ed.). Connecticut: Appleton and Lange.

Greenspan, F., & Strewler, G. (Eds). (1997) *Basic and clinical endocrinology* (5th ed.). Connecticut: Appleton & Lange.

Guyton, A. C., and Hall, J. E. (1996). *Textbook of medical physiology* (9th ed.). Philadelphia: Saunders.

Ignatavicius, D., & Bayne, M. (1991). *Medical-surgical. A nursing process approach.* Philadelphia: W. B. Saunders.

Kinney, M., Packa, D., & Dunbar, S. (1993). *AACN's clinical reference for critical-care nursing* (3rd ed.). St. Louis: C. V. Mosby.

McCance, K. L., & Huether, S. E. (1994). *Pathophysiology: The biologic basis for disease in adults and children* (2nd ed.). St. Louis: Mosby–Year Book.

Peragallo-Dittko, V. (1993). *Core curriculum for diabetes education* (2nd ed.). Chicago: American Association of Diabetes Educators.

Porth, C. (1994). *Pathophysiology: Concepts of altered health states* (4th ed.). Philadelphia: Lippincott-Raven.

Thelan, L., Davie, J., et al. (1994). *Critical care nursing diagnosis and management* (2nd ed.). St. Louis: C. V. Mosby.

Wilson, J. D. & Foster, D. W. (Eds). (1997) *Williams textbook of endocrinology* (9th ed.). Philadelphia: Saunders.

STUDY QUESTIONS

1. Phosphorus is primarily excreted via the:
   a. skin
   b. liver
   c. intestines
   d. kidneys

2. When providing patient teaching about phosphorus-rich foods, the nurse would not recommend:
   a. lettuce
   b. spinach
   c. broccoli
   d. cheese

3. Normal serum phosphorus concentration ranges from:
   a. 1.0 to 2.5 mEq/dL
   b. 2.5 to 4.5 mEq/dL
   c. 3.0 to 6.0 mEq/dL
   d. 5.0 to 9.5 mEq/dL

4. Conditions that result in osteoporosis may cause hyperphosphatemia because:
   a. Phosphorus is removed from the bone.
   b. Phosphorus replaces calcium in the bone.
   c. The medications used to treat osteoporosis may cause it.
   d. As calcium levels increase, so do phosphorus levels.

5. Symptoms of hypophosphatemia include all of the following except:
   a. hemolytic anemia
   b. muscle spasms
   c. positive Chvostek's sign
   d. positive Trousseau's sign

6. Phosphorus is necessary for:
   a. energy creation
   b. electrolyte diffusion
   c. normal urine function
   d. adequate cardiac contraction

7. Which one of the following endocrine hormones helps regulate phosphorus levels?
   a. antidiuretic hormone (ADH)
   b. adrenocorticotropic hormone (ACTH)
   c. parathyroid hormone (PTH)
   d. growth hormone (GH)

8. When caring for a patient with hyperphosphatemia, the nurse should be prepared to administer which of the following medications?
   a. Inderal
   b. Tagamet
   c. Dilantin
   d. Basaljel

9. A patient with renal related hyperphosphatemia must receive a phosphate binder along with:
   a. calcium binders
   b. potassium supplements
   c. calcium supplements
   d. magnesium supplements

10. A nurse administering a bowel prep with Fleet's Phospo-soda and other laxatives knows that which electrolyte imbalance can occur?
    a. hypercalcemia
    b. hypocalcemia
    c. hypophosphatemia
    d. hyperphosphatemia

ANSWER KEY

Question	Correct answer	Correct answer rationale	Incorrect answer rationales
1.	d	Phosphorus is excreted via the kidneys; renal failure can result in hyperphosphatemia.	a, b, and c. These responses are incorrect.
2.	d	Dairy products are rich in phosphorous.	a, b, and c. Green, leafy vegetables are not rich in phosphorus.
3.	b	Normal serum phosphorus concentration ranges from 2.5 to 4.5 mEq/dl.	a, c, and d. These values do not reflect normal levels.
4.	a	As calcium is lost from the bone, so too will phosphorus be lost.	b, c, and d. These responses are incorrect.
5.	a	Hemolytic anemia occurs with hypophosphatemia because phosphorous is essential to the functioning of red blood cells, and these cells are easily destroyed in the presence of hypophosphatemia.	b, c, and d. Positive Chvostek's, Trousseau's sign, and muscle spasms are found in hyperphosphatemia.
6.	a	Phosphorus is necessary for the creation of energy through cellular metabolism, where adenosine triphosphate (ATP) is enzymatically split to produce phosphate and energy.	b. Phosphorus is required to maintain normal cell membrane integrity, but it is not directly responsible for diffusion. c. Phosphorus levels do not affect urinary system functioning. d. Although phosphorus is an intracellular electrolyte, it does not affect cardiac contraction.
7.	c	Parathyroid hormone (PTH) regulates phosphorus levels by its response to calcium, which then affects phosphorus. When calcium levels decrease, PTH is secreted, moving calcium from bone to serum. The presence of PTH inhibits tubular reabsorption of phosphorus, allowing more phosphorus to be excreted.	a, b, and d. These hormones do not influence phosphorus levels.
8.	d	Basalgel is a phosphate-binding medication; its use allows dietary phosphorus to be bound in the gut and excreted.	a, b, and c. These drugs do not not affect phosphorus levels.
9.	c	In the presence of renal failure calcium supplements must be given with phosphate binders.	a, b, and d. These are not appropriate interventions . for the situations described
10.	d	Hyperphosphatemia, not hypophosphatemia (letter c), is possible because these preparations are high in phosphorous.	a and b. Calcium levels are not effected by these preparations.

Acid–Base Balance

I. Overview of acids and bases

A. Description
   1. *Acids* are substances that can release hydrogen ions.
   2. *Bases* (alkalis) are substances that can accept hydrogen ions; bases include bicarbonate (HCO_3) ions.

   3. **Carbon dioxide (CO_2) is considered to be an acid or a base depending on its chemical association. When assessing acid–base balance, it is considered an acid because of its relationship with carbonic acid (H_2CO_3). Because carbonic acid cannot be measured, CO_2 measures are used.**
   4. To maintain the balance between acids and bases, dynamic processes continually adjust the concentration of hydrogen ions (H^+) and hydroxide ions (OH^-) within body fluids.
   5. A measure of the ratio between acids and bases or the concentration of hydrogen ions within body fluids is known as the percent of hydrogen ions in solution (pH).

   6. **Normal values for blood pH range within a narrow margin:**
      a. **Normal values for arterial blood range from 7.35 to 7.45.**
      b. **Extreme high and low pH values (such as 6.8 or 7.8) are incompatible with life.**
   7. An abnormal increase in hydrogen ions or decrease in bicarbonate ions re-

sults in *acidosis;* pH values drop below 7.35. An abnormal decrease in hydrogen ions or increase in bicarbonate ions results in *alkalosis;* pH values increase above 7.45. (See Chapter 12, Alterations in Acid–Base Balance, for more information.)

    8. *Buffers* are chemicals that maintain pH by ensuring a stable hydrogen ion concentration.

B. **Supply and sources**

    1. Acids and bases are found in:
- a. Extracellular fluid (ECF)
- b. Intracellular fluid (ICF)
- c. Body tissues

    2. Foods can produce acids and bases as a result of metabolism:
- a. Meats provide a dietary source of acids; meat is the main metabolic source of hydrogen ions.
- b. Fruits provide a dietary source of bases.
- c. Vegetables can provide acids and bases.

    3. Certain activities or conditions that are characterized by fat metabolism (eg, strenuous exercise and states of starvation) can produce acids.

    4. Catabolic processes also are known to release organic acids into the ECF.

    5. CO_2 is produced as an acid and a base by normal cellular metabolism.

C. **Role**

    1. Assist in maintaining a stable concentration of hydrogen ions in body fluids

    2. Maintain pH and thereby provide the necessary environment for bodily functions (eg, cellular metabolism and enzymatic processes) to occur

    3. Provide a neutral environment

    4. Compensate for specific imbalances

II.   Acid–base balance

A. **Description**

    1. Acids are constantly being produced through bodily functions and processes.

    2. Balancing acids and bases requires acids to be neutralized or excreted.

    3. CO_2, an acid, and HCO_3, a base, are crucial in maintaining acid–base balance.

    4. Normally, acid–base balance is maintained when the ratio of bicarbonate (HCO_3) to carbonic acid (H_2CO_3) is 20 to 1. (Note that carbonic acid is measured by carbon dioxide.)

B. **Acid–base balance measurement**

    1. Arterial blood gas (ABG) values are used to measure acid–base balance (Table 11-1).

     2. **ABG values show:**
- a. **The amount of oxygen (O_2), a gas, in the serum**
- b. **The amount of carbon dioxide (CO_2), a gas, in the serum**
- c. **The pH, or percentage of hydrogen ions, in solution**

    3. ABG analysis reveals:
- a. If the patient has enough O_2 to maintain perfusion

TABLE 11-1
Arterial Blood Gases

TERM	NORMAL VALUE	DEFINITION-IMPLICATIONS
pH	7.35–7.45	Reflects H^+ concentration; acidity increases as H^+ concentration increases (pH value decreases as acidity increases) • pH <7.35 (acidosis) • pH >7.45 (alkalosis)
$PaCO_2$	35–45 mmHg	Partial pressure of CO_2 in arterial blood • When <35 mmHg, hypocapnia is said to be present (respiratory alkalosis) • When >45 mmHg, hypercapnia is said to be present (respiratory alkalosis)
PaO_2	80–100 mmHg	Partial pressure of O_2 in arterial blood
Standard HCO_3	22–26 mEq/L	HCO_3 concentration in plasma of blood that has been equilibrated at a $PaCO_2$ of 40 mmHg, and with O_2 to fully saturate the hemoglobin

Metheny, N. M. (1996). Fluid and electrolyte balance (3rd ed.) Philadelphia: Lippincott-Raven, p. 161.

    b.   If enough CO_2 is being eliminated
    c.   The ratio of hydrogen to bicarbonate

III.   Acid–base regulation

A.   Chemical buffer system

1. Chemical buffers are present in all body fluids (ICF and ECF), tissue, and bone.
2. The chemical buffer system functions primarily to maintain a constant serum pH; to do this, buffers continually accept or release free hydrogen ions.
3. The three major buffer systems include:
   a. Carbonic acid–bicarbonate buffer system
   b. Phosphate buffer system
   c. Protein buffer system
4. The *carbonic acid–bicarbonate buffer system* is the primary ECF buffer. It is characterized by a series of chemical reactions between carbonic acid (H_2CO_3) and bicarbonate (HCO_3).
5. The *phosphate buffer system* buffers the ICF and ECF. A series of chemical reactions between buffering salts and hydrogen ions work to maintain pH.
6. The *protein buffer system* is a powerful and abundant ICF buffer. It works similarly to the carbonic acid–bicarbonate buffer system.
7. Bone buffers also can contribute to the buffering of acids and bases.
8. All of the chemical buffer systems work interdependently and require respiratory and renal regulation as well to maintain acid–base balance.
9. Table 11-2 provides more information about the chemical buffer system.

TABLE 11-2
Chemical Buffer System

Carbonic Acid–Bicarbonate Buffer System	Handles more than 50% of all chemical buffer activities
	Takes place in body fluids and renal tubules
	Is illustrated by the following chemical expression:
	$CO_2 + H_2O \leftrightarrow H_2CO_3 \leftrightarrow H^+ + HCO_3^-$
	Involves Na, K, Ca, Cl, and Mg when changes in the chemical buffering system are underway, thereby affecting pH, acid–base balance, and electrolyte balance
Phosphate Buffer System	Takes place in body fluids and renal tubules
	Provides important buffering effects in the kidney's tubular fluid
	Results in pH adjustments through the reactions of dihydrogen phosphate ions and monohydrogen phosphate ions with acids or bases
	Is important in maintaining urine pH
Protein Buffer System	Performs the majority of ICF buffering
	Takes place inside the cells
	Works similarly to carbonic acid–bicarbonate buffer system
	Uses hemoglobin, which acts as an immediate protein buffer for volatile acids
Bone Buffer System	Takes place in bone and ECF
	Increases the use of bone carbonate when CRF is present; chronic buffering by bone is, in part, an etiology for various bone diseases occurring with CRF

ICF, intracellular fluid; ECF, extracellular fluid; CRF, chronic renal failure

B. Respiratory regulation

1. The respiratory center in the medulla and the lungs is involved in respiratory regulation and compensation of the acid–base balance.

2. The lungs use carbon dioxide (CO_2) to regulate hydrogen ion concentration.

 3. **Through changes in the rate and depth of respirations, acid–base balance is achieved through CO_2 elimination or retention.**

4. Hypoventilation causes retention of acids as CO_2 is retained; hyperventilation causes alkalosis as CO_2 is rapidly eliminated through the increased respiration.

5. This respiratory regulation process occurs within minutes.

6. Changes in respiratory status for any reason can lead to changes in pH.

7. Compensation occurs in response to metabolic disturbances.

8. When there is excessive hydrogen ions present, the medullary chemoreceptors stimulate increased respirations in an attempt to blow off the excess acids as CO_2; excessive bases are sensed in the medulla and the respirations decrease. The acid CO_2 will then be retained and balance with the excess bases will be present.

9. This occurs within minutes but is only a temporary or limited response.

TABLE 11-3
Renal Regulation

Bicarbonate Reabsorption	Secreted hydrogen ions combine with bicarbonate to form carbonic acid. Carbonic anhydrase reacts with carbonic acid to form water and carbon dioxide. The water is excreted, and the carbon dioxide diffuses to the tubular cells. Carbonic anhydrase reacts with carbon dioxide to form bicarbonate, which can be reabsorbed by the proximal tubules and returned to body fluids.
Bicarbonate Production	Hydrogen ions are secreted. Carbonic acid dissociates into hydrogen ions and bicarbonate. Hydrogen ions are excreted. Bicarbonate moves to the peritubular capillary.
Hydrogen Ion Excretion	Ammonia (NH_3) combines with hydrogen ions to form ammonium (NH_4). NH_4 cannot cross cell membranes and is excreted. Similar excretion of hydrogen ions is achieved with phosphates and titratable acids.

C. Renal regulation

1. **Renal regulation of acid–base balance (Table 11-3) is achieved by three interrelated processes:**
   a. **Bicarbonate reabsorption**
   b. **Bicarbonate formation**
   c. **Hydrogen ion excretion**
2. *Bicarbonate reabsorption* occurs in the proximal tubule; it requires secretion of hydrogen ions by the kidneys and the enzymatic action of carbonic anhydrase. The reabsorbed bicarbonate is returned to body fluids, where it is available for the chemical buffer system.
3. *Bicarbonate production* is needed to replace the bicarbonate that has been used to maintain the bicarbonate concentration; this is done by the kidneys. Bicarbonate produced by the kidneys increases the plasma concentration.
4. The production of bicarbonate also involves secreting hydrogen ions.
5. Hydrogen ions accumulate from dietary, metabolic, and secretory sources.
6. *Hydrogen ion excretion* helps maintain acid–base balance. When excessive amounts of hydrogen are present, the volume delivered to the kidneys is high, creating an acidic glomerular filtrate and subsequently acidic urine.
7. Hydrogen ions also are excreted after they are buffered with ammonia.
8. Compensation for metabolic disturbances in acid–base balance is provided by the kidneys.

Bibliography

Bullock, B. (1996). *Pathophysiology: Adaptations and alterations in function* (4th ed.). Philadelphia: J. B. Lippincott.

Drummer, C., Gerzer, R., Heer, M., et al. (1992). Effects of an acute saline infusion on fluid and electrolyte metabolism in humans. *American Journal of Physiology,* May, 744–754.

Guyton, A. (1991). *Textbook of medical physiology* (8th ed.). Philadelphia: W. B. Saunders.

Kinney, M., Packa, D., & Dunbar, S. (1993). *AACN's clinical reference for critical-care nursing* (3rd ed.). St. Louis: C.V. Mosby.

Kokko, J., & Tannen, R. (1996). *Fluids and electrolytes* (3rd ed.). Philadelphia: W. B. Saunders.

Metheny, N. (1996). *Fluid and electrolyte balance: Nursing considerations* (3rd ed.). Philadelphia: J. B. Lippincott.

Miller, M. (1997). Fluid and electrolyte homeostasis in the elderly: physiologic changes of aging and clinical consequences. *Baillieres Clinical Endocrinology and Metabolism,* 11(2), 367–387.

Narrins, R. (Ed). (1994). *Maxwell & Kleemans clinical disorders of fluid and electrolyte metabolism* (5th ed.). New York: McGraw-Hill.

North American Nursing Diagnosis Association. Nursing Diagnosis: Definitions and Classifications. The Auth. 1996.

Plante, G. E., Chakir, M., Lehoux, S., & Lortie, M. (1995). Disorders of body fluid balance: A new look into the mechanisms of disease. *Canadian Journal of Cardiology,* 11(9), 788–802.

Porth, C. (1994). *Pathophysiology: Concepts of altered health states* (4th ed.). Philadelphia: J. B. Lippincott.

Rose, B. (1994). *Clinical physiology of acid-base and electrolyte disorders* (4th ed.). New York: McGraw-Hill.

Seaman, S. L. (1995). Renal physiology part II: Fluid and electrolyte regulation. *Neonatal network,* 14(5), 5–11.

Smith, K., & Brain, E. (1991). *Fluids and electrolytes: A conceptual approach* (2nd ed.). New York: Churchill Livingstone.

Szerlip, H., & Goldfarb, S. (1993). *Workshops in fluid and electrolyte disorders.* New York: Churchill Livingstone.

Toto, K. (1994). Endocrine physiology. *Critical Care Nursing Clinics of North America,* December, 647–657.

STUDY QUESTIONS

1. Which of the following systems is *not* involved in maintaining acid–base balance except?
   a. respiratory
   b. chemical
   c. blood
   d. renal

2. Normal values for arterial blood pH range from:
   a. 7.31 to 7.41
   b. 7.35 to 7.45
   c. 6.8 to 7.8
   d. 7.5 to 8.0

3. Balancing acids and bases requires neutralizing or excreting of acids because:
   a. Acids are stronger than bases.
   b. The body is constantly producing acids through body functions and processes.
   c. All foods produce acids.
   d. Acids are toxic to body tissues.

4. Chemical buffers function to:
   a. Maintain a constant serum pH.
   b. Accept or release free hydroxide ions.
   c. Remain dormant until needed to rebalance acid and bases.
   d. Eliminate or retain CO_2 to maintain balance.

5. When assessing acid–base balance, the nurse would consider which of the following to be an acid?
   a. carbon dioxide
   b. sodium bicarbonate
   c. oxygen
   d. calcium phosphate

6. A nurse caring for a patient who is in a state of excessive catabolism (accelerated breakdown of proteins) knows that this patient may be at risk for:
   a. alkalosis
   b. acidosis
   c. hypoxia
   d. hypercapnia

7. Which of the following conditions may produce acids?
   a. resting
   b. overeating
   c. starvation
   d. obesity

8. Which is the primary extracellular fluid (ECF) buffer system?
   a. phosphate buffer system
   b. carbonic acid buffer system
   c. protein buffer system
   d. ammonia buffer system

9. Renal regulation of acids and bases occurs by:
   a. bicarbonate excretion
   b. hydrogen reabsorption
   c. hydrogen formation
   d. hydrogen excretion

10. The respiratory system compensates for metabolic alkalosis by:
    a. increasing sputum production
    b. increasing respirations
    c. decreasing respirations
    d. decreasing respiratory depth

ANSWER KEY

Question	Correct answer	Correct answer rationale	Incorrect answer rationales
1.	c	Blood is not one of the regulation systems involved in maintaining acid–base balance.	a, b, and d. The respiratory, chemical, and renal systems are involved in maintaining the body's acid–base balance.
2.	b	Normal arterial pH, a measure of the ratio between acids and bases, ranges from 7.35 to 7.45.	a, c, and d. These are not normal blood gas ranges.
3.	b	The body is constantly producing acids through body functions and processes. Balancing acids and bases requires neutralization or excretion of acids.	a, c, and d. These are not true statements.
4.	a	Chemical buffers function to accept or release free hydrogen ions in an attempt to maintain acid–base balance and a normal pH.	b. Chemical buffers accept or release hydrogen ions, not hydroxide ions. c. Chemical buffers are constantly in action. d. Buffers do not eliminate.
5.	a	When assessing acid–base balance, carbon dioxide is considered to be an acid because of its relationship with carbonic acid (H_2CO_3).	b and d. These are not considered in the arterial blood gas (ABG) assessment. c. This response is not an acid.
6.	b	Catabolic processes are known to release organic acids into the ECF.	a, c, and d. These conditions may be revealed by ABG assessment, but are not related to catabolism.
7.	c	Starvation causes fat metabolism, which results in the liberation of acids.	a, b, and d. Resting, overeating, and obesity have no effect on acid production.
8.	b	The carbonic acid–bicarbonate buffer system is the primary ECF buffer. It is characterized by a series of chemical reactions between carbonic acid and bicarbonate.	a. Although the phosphate buffer system works in the ECF and ICF, it remains secondary to the carbonic acid–bicarbonate buffer system. c and d. These buffer systems are secondary to the carbonic acid–bicarbonate buffer system and work in the intracellular space.
9.	d	Renal regulation occurs through bicarbonate reabsorption, bicarbonate formation, hydrogen ion secretion.	a, b, and c. See above.
10.	b	The lungs compensate for metabolic alkalosis by hyperventilation. This allows the lungs to "blow off" the excess CO_2.	a, c, and d. These do not describe compensatory mechanisms for metabolic alkalosis.

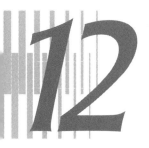

Alterations in
Acid–Base Balance

I. Introduction

A. Overview

1. **Acid–base balance is necessary to maintain homeostasis in the body's fluids.**

2. Alterations in acid–base balance result in changes in certain bodily functions (eg, respiratory stimulation, maintenance of electrolyte balance).

3. *Acidosis* refers to an abnormal increase in hydrogen ions or decrease in bicarbonate ions.

4. *Alkalosis* refers to an abnormal decrease in hydrogen ions or increase in bicarbonate ions.

123

DISPLAY 12-1
Anion Gap Metabolic Acidosis

- Anion gap refers to the difference between anions and cations in the ECF; it can be calculated as follows:
  anion gap = $Na - (Cl + HCO_3) = 12 \pm 2$ mEq/L
  (The difference between anions and cations must equal 12 [plus or minus 2].)
- When an anion gap is greater than 12, the ratio of anions to cations is increased, setting homeostatic mechanisms off balance and resulting in acidosis. The higher the gap, the worse the acidosis.
- Conditions that cause anion gap acidosis include *diabetic ketoacidosis* (in which ketones are produced in large amounts), *lactic acidosis* (in which excess lactic acid is produced due to poor tissue perfusion), and *salicylate intoxication* (due to the highly acidic metabolites produced by salicylate breakdown).

B. **Types of acid–base imbalances**

    1. Single acid–base imbalances include:

        a. Respiratory acidosis

        b. Respiratory alkalosis

        c. Metabolic acidosis

        d. Metabolic alkalosis

    2. Metabolic acidosis may be classified into two types:

        a. Nonanion gap acidosis

        b. Anion gap acidosis, which is uncommon (see Display 12-1 for more information)

    3. Mixed acid–base disorders occur when two or more single acid–base imbalances are present, causing arterial blood gas (ABG) abnormalities:

        a. To determine whether these changed ABG values relate to compensation or represent the emergence of a second acid–base imbalance, the nurse must conduct a careful assessment. (Display 12-2 outlines the necessary steps in the ABG assessment.)

        b. Clinical conditions associated with mixed acid–base imbalances include cardiopulmonary distress, renal failure with gastric drainage and vomiting, renal failure with chronic obstructive pulmonary disease (COPD), COPD with vomiting, and renal failure with pneumonia. Any coexisting respiratory disorder can yield a mixed acid–base disorder.

II. Respiratory acidosis

A. **Description**

    1. **Respiratory acidosis is an acid–base imbalance caused by a decrease in pulmonary ventilation (eg, hypoventilation).**

    2. Hypoventilation increases carbon dioxide (CO_2) concentration in the lungs and blood.

    3. Increased carbon dioxide concentration increases the level of carbonic acid (H_2CO_2) and hydrogen ions circulating in the blood, lowering arterial pH levels toward 7.0.

DISPLAY 12-2
Systematic Assessment of Arterial Blood Gases

The following steps are recommended to evaluate arterial blood gas values. They are based on the assumption that the average values are

$$pH = 7.4$$
$$PaCO_2 = 40 \text{ mm Hg}$$
$$HCO_3 = 24 \text{ mEq/L}$$

I. *First*, look at the pH. It can be high, low, or normal as follows:

$$pH > 7.4 \text{ (alkalosis)}$$
$$pH < 7.4 \text{ (acidosis)}$$
$$pH = 7.4 \text{ (normal)}$$

A normal pH may indicate prefectly normal blood gases, or it may be an indication of a *compensated* imbalance. A compensated imbalance is one in which the body has been able to correct the pH by either respiratory or metaoblic changes (depending on the primary problem). For example, a patient with primary metabolic acidosis starts out with a low bicarbonate level but a normal carbon dioxide level. Soon afterward, the lungs try to compensate for the imbalance by exhaling large amounts of carbon dioxide (hyperventilation). Another example, a patient with primary respiratory acidosis starts out with a high carbon dioxide level; soon afterward, the kidneys attempt to compensate by retaining bicarbonate. If the compensatory maneuver is able to restore the bicarbonate: carbonic acid ratio back to 20: 1, full compensation (and thus normal pH) will be achieved.

II. *The next step is to determine the primary cause of the disturbance. This is done by evaluating the PaCO$_2$ and HCO$_3$ in relation to the pH.*
   pH > 7.4 (alkalosis)
   1. *If the PaCO$_2$ is < 40 mm Hg*, the primary disturbance is respiratory alkalosis. (This situation occurs when a patient hyperventilates and "blows off" too much carbon dioxide. Recall that carbon dioxide dissolved in water becomes carbonic acid, the acid side of the "carbonic acid : base bicarbonate" buffer system.)
   2. *If the HCO$_3$ is > 24 mEq/L*, the primary disturbance is metabolic alkalosis. (This situation occurs when the body gains too much bicarbonate, an alkaline substance. Bicarbonate is the basic, or alkaline side of the "carbonic acid–base : bicarbonate buffer system.")
   pH < 7.4 (acidosis)
   1. *If the PaCO$_2$ is > 40 mm Hg*, the primary disturbance is respiratory acidosis. (This situation occurs when a patient hypoventilates and thus retains too much carbon dioxide, an acidic substance.)
   2. *If the HCO$_3$ is < 24 mEq/L*, the primary disturbance is metabolic acidosis. (This situation occurs when the body's bicarbonate level drops, either because of direct bicarbonate loss or because of gains of acids such as lactic acid or ketones).

III. *The next step involves determining if compensation has begun.*
   This is done by looking at the value other than the primary disorder. If it is moving in the same direction as the primary value, compensation is underway. Consider the following gases:
   Example:

pH	PaCO$_2$	HCO$_3$
(1) 7.20	60 mm Hg	24 mEq/L
(2) 7.40	60 mm Hg	37 mEq/L

   The first set (1) indicates acute respiratory acidosis without compensation (the PaCO$_2$ is high, the HcO$_3$ is normal). The second set (2) indicates chronic respiratory acidosis. Note that compensation has taken place; that is, the HCO$_3$ has elevated to an appropriate level to balance the high PaCO$_2$ and produce a normal pH.

(Source: Metheny, N. M. (1996). Fluid and electrolyte balance (3rd ed.). Philadelphia: Lippincott-Raven.)

4. The body tries to restore normal pH by a process called compensation, which occurs in the kidneys:
    a. Compensation is achieved by reducing the amount of bicarbonate (HCO_3) ions excreted in the kidney.
    b. This occurs through increased renal absorption of bicarbonate.

B.   Etiology

1. **Any factor that interferes with the exchange of gases between blood and air present in alveolus can result in respiratory acidosis. These causes can be acute or chronic, but all are related to a state of hypoventilation.**
2. Acute causes include:
    a. Cardiopulmonary arrest
    b. Pneumothorax or hydrothorax
    c. Chest wall trauma
    d. Acute abdominal distention
    e. Drug overdose (eg, sedatives, anesthesia)
    f. Airway obstruction
    g. Pulmonary edema
    h. Atelectasis
    i. Pneumonia
    j. Acute neurologic dysfunction from any cause (eg, cerebral trauma, Guillain-Barré syndrome).
3. Chronic causes include:
    a. Chronic emphysema and bronchitis
    b. Myasthenia gravis
    c. Cystic fibrosis
    d. COPD
    e. Congestive heart failure
    f. Pulmonary fibrosis

C.   Assessment findings

1. Symptoms result as acids accumulate and serum pH decreases; as the pH level drops, symptoms progress in severity.
2. Symptoms can include:
    a. Tachycardia
    b. Dyspnea
    c. Slow, shallow respirations
    d. Tremors
    e. Confusion
    f. Dizziness
    g. Asterixis
    h. Altered level of consciousness
    i. Convulsions
    j. Warm, flushed skin
    k. Cyanosis
3. Laboratory findings in respiratory acidosis reveal alterations in normal ABG values for pH and $PaCO_2$ (Table 12-1):
    a. The pH is below 7.35; the lower the pH, the more severe the acidosis.

TABLE 12-1
Acid–Base Imbalances: Arterial Blood Gas Analysis

DISORDER	pH	PaCO$_2$	HCO$_3$
Respiratory acidosis (uncompensated)	Below 7.35	Above 42	Normal
Respiratory acidosis (partially uncompensated)	Below 7.35	Above 42	Above 26 (Bicarbonate is retained to buffer the acid [CO$_2$] and move the pH to normal.)
Respiratory acidosis (fully compensated)	Normal	Above 42	Above 26
Respiratory alkalosis (uncompensated)	Above 7.45	Below 38	Normal
Respiratory alkalosis (partially compensated)	Above 7.45	Below 38	Below 22 (The kidneys eliminate bicarbonate to balance with the lowered acid levels, moving the pH toward normal.)
Respiratory alkalosis (fully compensated)	Normal	Below 38	Below 22
Metabolic acidosis (uncompensated)	Below 7.35	Normal	Below 22
Metabolic acidosis (partially compensated)	Below 7.35	Below 38	Below 22 (The respiratory system responds by hyperventilating, which eliminates the acid CO$_2$ in an attempt to eliminate extra acids and move the pH toward normal.)
Metabolic acidosis (fully compensated)	Normal	Below 38	Below 22
Metabolic alkalosis (uncompensated)	Above 7.45	Normal	Above 26
Metabolic alkalosis (partially compensated)	Above 7.45	Above 42	Above 26 (The respiratory system responds by hypoventilating to retain more acid so that the extra bicarbonate will be buffered, moving the pH toward normal.)
Metabolic alkalosis (fully compensated)	Normal	Above 42	Above 26

       b. PaCO$_2$ is above 42, indicating acids (CO$_2$) are being retained and that this is the cause of decreased pH.

       c. HCO$_3$ is normal, indicating that there is no metabolic component.

   4. **As renal compensation occurs, the pH moves closer to normal. Increasing levels of bicarbonate (due to renal absorption of bicarbonate) move the pH in a normal direction.**

    5. ABG results reveal the level of compensation at the time the specimen is taken; a normal pH indicates full compensation.

D. **Potential nursing diagnoses**

    1. Activity Intolerance

    2. Ineffective Breathing Pattern

3. Altered Tissue Perfusion
4. Impaired Memory
5. Risk for Injury
6. Ineffective Breathing Pattern
7. Impaired Verbal Communication
8. Fatigue
9. Altered Thought Process

E.   Interventions
1. Plan the patient's activities to allow for rest intervals.
2. Keep needed objects within the patient's easy reach.
3. Position the patient in semi-Fowler's position to ease the work of breathing.
4. Encourage deep breathing, coughing, and changes in position at least every 2 hours.
5. Institute chest physiotherapy.
6. Suction airway to maintain patency.
7. Provide emotional support and reassurance to allay anxiety.
8. Monitor respiratory rate and depth frequently depending on each case.
9. Administer low flow oxygen therapy as ordered.
10. Monitor ABG levels for changes in pH and CO_2.
11. Force fluids (2 to 3 L daily, unless contraindicated) to loosen secretions and aid in expectoration.

F.   Evaluation
1. Normal exchange of oxygen and carbon dioxide occurs.
2. The patient achieves maximum ventilation.
3. The patient reports no dyspnea.
4. ABG values return to normal ranges.

III.   Respiratory alkalosis

A.   Description

1. **Respiratory alkalosis is an acid–base imbalance caused by an increase in the pulmonary ventilation rate (eg, hyperventilation).**
2. Hyperventilation decreases serum carbon dioxide in the lungs and blood as carbon dioxide is eliminated with the excess respirations. (The ratio of CO_2 to bicarbonate then changes, with bicarbonate being excessive due to a loss of CO_2.)
3. Decreased carbon dioxide concentration decreases the level of carbonic acid (H_2CO_3) and hydrogen ions circulating in the blood, raising arterial pH levels.
4. The body tries to restore the pH to normal through renal compensation; in this process, renal excretion of bicarbonate is increased.

B.   Etiology
1. Any factor that contributes to hyperventilation, which lowers $PaCO_2$, can cause respiratory alkalosis.
2. Potential causes include:
   a. Acute hypoxia (eg, due to pneumonia, asthma, pulmonary edema)

    b. Chronic hypoxia (eg, due to pulmonary fibrosis, cyanotic heart disease, high altitudes)
    c. Anxiety
    d. Fever
    e. Aspirin overdose
    f. Central nervous system trauma or seizures
    g. Exercise
    h. Gram-negative sepsis
    i. Hepatic cirrhosis
    j. Excessive mechanical ventilation
    k. Pregnancy

C. Assessment findings

   1. Symptoms result as acids are reduced and bicarbonate accumulates; symptoms may include:
    a. Paresthesia
    b. Numbness and tingling
    c. Light-headedness
    d. Confusion
    e. Tetany and loss of consciousness (if alkalosis is severe)

   2. Laboratory findings reveal alterations in normal ABG values for pH and $PaCO_2$ (see Table 12-1):
    a. The pH is above 7.45; the higher the pH, the worse the alkalosis.
    b. $PaCO_2$ is below 38, indicating a loss of the acid CO_2.
    c. HCO_3 is normal, making the ratio of acids to bases excessive on the base side; a normal bicarbonate indicates that there is no metabolic compensation.

   3. As renal compensation occurs, the pH moves closer to normal as bicarbonate is excreted by the kidneys. A normal pH indicates full compensation.

D. Potential nursing diagnoses

   1. Ineffective Breathing Pattern
   2. High Risk for Injury
   3. Anxiety
   4. Impaired Memory
   5. Fatigue
   6. Activity Intolerance
   7. Altered Thought Process

E. Interventions

   1. Assist in achieving the goal of reducing the ventilation rate or maintaining the balance.
   2. Encourage slow, deep breathing (use a paper bag or rebreathing mask, if necessary).
   3. Monitor vital signs, especially respiratory rate and depth.
   4. If sedation is used to slow respiratory rate, assess the patient for respiratory depression.
   5. Provide emotional support and reassurance to the patient to reduce anxiety.
   6. Institute and maintain seizure precautions.
   7. Assist the patient with activities of daily living.

F.   Evaluation

  1.   The patient remains free from injury.
  2.   The patient displays regular respiratory rate and breathing pattern.
  3.   ABG values return to normal ranges.

IV.   Metabolic acidosis

A.   Description

  1.   **Metabolic acidosis is an acid–base imbalance caused by an increased accumulation of metabolic acids (eg, lactic acid and ketoacids) that rise in proportion to bicarbonate, resulting in decreased arterial pH.**
  2.   Electrolytes always compete with each other for binding. In instances of metabolic acidosis, chloride and bicarbonate compete to bind with sodium. Acidosis also allows more chloride to be present, accounting for increased acids.
  3.   A loss of bicarbonate ions (bases) also causes acidosis because the acid–base balance is offset by the greater amount of acids present.
  4.   As the pH decreases with rising levels of acids (as compared with bicarbonate), the excess hydrogen ions stimulate chemoreceptors.
  5.   The chemoreceptors in turn increase the respiratory rate (hyperventilation), causing respiratory compensation. This occurs immediately at the onset of acidosis.
  6.   Hyperventilation occurs to compensate and lower the CO_2 levels, moving the ratio of CO_2 to H_2CO_3 toward normal.
  7.   After several hours of respiratory compensation, the pH returns to a range between 7.35 and 7.45.
  8.   Even though the respiratory system compensates, the underlying metabolic disturbance may still remain.

B.   Etiology

  1.   Metabolic acid build-up occurs when:
      a.   Metabolic demands are greater than carbohydrate stores or when carbohydrates are not used normally by body cells, resulting in fat metabolism (eg, ketoacidosis or starvation).
      b.   Metabolism occurs anaerobically (lactic acidosis).
      c.   The kidneys are unable to retain bicarbonate (eg, renal failure).
  2.   Other causes of metabolic acidosis include:
      a.   Salicylate toxicity
      b.   Loss of bicarbonate through the renal system (diuretics) or gastrointestinal system (diarrhea)
      c.   Trauma or burns in which lactic acid is produced (due to lack of oxygen availability to the cells)

C.   Assessment findings

  1.   Symptoms result as acids accumulate, changing the levels of other electrolytes, and as compensation occurs; symptoms may include:
      a.   Kussmaul's respirations
      b.   Fruity breath (when diabetic ketoacidosis is the cause)
      c.   Lethargy
      d.   Drowsiness

       e. Confusion
       f. Headache
       g. Stupor
       h. Seizures
       i. Twitching
       j. Nausea
       k. Vomiting
       l. Peripheral vasodilation
       m. Flushed skin
       n. Warm, dry skin
       o. Hyperkalemia or hyperchloremia (possible)

  2. Laboratory results reveal alterations in normal ABG values for pH and HCO_3 (see Table 12-1):

       a. The pH is below 7.35; the lower the pH, the more severe the acidosis.
       b. $PaCO_2$ is normal.
       c. HCO_3 is lowered.

  3. A normal $PaCO_2$ indicates that respiratory compensation has not occurred.

  4. Compensation occurs as the respiratory system increases its ventilation rate to blow off more acids (CO_2) in an attempt to eliminate excess acid and move the pH toward normal.

  5. A normal pH indicates full compensation.

D. Potential nursing diagnoses

  1. Risk for Injury
  2. Altered Tissue Perfusion
  3. Altered Nutrition: More Than Body Requirements
  4. Anxiety
  5. Altered Thought Process

E. Interventions

  1. Institute and maintain safety precautions (eg, side rails, seizure precautions).
  2. Monitor hemodynamic status through blood pressure and pulse rate and rhythm.
  3. Assess peripheral vascular status (eg, capillary refill, temperature, color).
  4. Monitor cardiac status.

F. Evaluation

  1. ABG values return to normal.
  2. Heart rate, rhythm, and blood pressure return to normal.
  3. The patient remains injury free.

V. Metabolic alkalosis

A. Description

  1. Metabolic alkalosis is an acid–base imbalance caused by an increased loss of acid (most often from the stomach or kidneys).

  2. Loss of a fixed acid decreases the hydrogen ion concentration.

  3. As the hydrogen ion concentration decreases, more carbonic acid breaks down, and serum bicarbonate concentration increases (because more concentration is available, the kidney reabsorbs more). This results in increased excretion of the cations hydrogen, potassium, and chloride.

4. Because chloride and bicarbonate compete with each other for sodium binding, as chloride levels drop through binding, bicarbonate levels rise in compensation to balance the sodium.

5. As a result, chemoreceptor stimulation is decreased, lowering the respiratory rate.

6. Hypoventilation, the respiratory compensatory mechanism, keeps more acids in the body to balance the excess bicarbonate.

7. This occurs as hypoventilation reduces the amount of CO_2 that is eliminated, allowing more CO_2 (an acid) to be reabsorbed.

B. Etiology

1. Vomiting or gastric drainage
2. Diuretic therapy
3. Posthypercapnia alkalosis
4. Cushing's syndrome
5. Primary aldosteronism
6. Bartter's syndrome
7. Severe potassium depletion

C. Assessment findings

1. Symptoms may include:
   a. Apathy
   b. Confusion
   c. Stupor
   d. Tetany (if serum calcium is borderline low)
   e. Decreased respiratory rate and depth (may be a compensatory mechanism to conserve CO_2)
   f. Dizziness
   g. Paresthesia (in fingers and toes)
   h. Carpopedal spasm
   i. Nausea and vomiting
   j. Seizures
   k. Low serum potassium and chloride levels (related to sodium levels)
   l. Electrocardiogram changes (alterations in T and U waves may occur due to hypokalemia)
   m. Urine pH less than 7.0 (occurs in patients with sustained metabolic alkalosis because the serum delivered to the tubules is rich in bicarbonate, resulting in bicarbonate secretion)

2. Laboratory test results reveal alterations in normal ABG values for pH and HCO_3 (see Table 12-1):
   a. The pH is above 7.45; the higher the pH, the worse the alkalosis.
   b. PCO_2 is normal.
   c. HCO_3 levels are higher, indicating that the cause is metabolic.

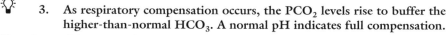 3. **As respiratory compensation occurs, the PCO_2 levels rise to buffer the higher-than-normal HCO_3. A normal pH indicates full compensation.**

D. Potential nursing diagnoses

1. Ineffective Breathing Patterns
2. High Risk for Injury

3.   Impaired Thought Process
4.   Anxiety
E.   Interventions
1.   Monitor respiratory rate and pattern.
2.   Auscultate lung sounds.
3.   Ensure adequate hydration.
4.   Monitor intake and output.
5.   Monitor serum electrolytes.
F.   Evaluation
1.   ABG and electrolyte values return to normal ranges.
2.   The patient's breathing patterns are normal.
3.   The patient is free from injury.

Bibliography

Bullock, B. (1996). *Pathophysiology: Adaptations and alterations in function* (4th ed.). Philadelphia: J. B. Lippincott.

Drummer, C., Gerzer, R., Heer, M., et al. (1992). Effects of an acute saline infusion on fluid and electrolyte metabolism in humans. *American Journal of Physiology,* May, 744–754.

Guyton, A. (1991). *Textbook of medical physiology* (8th ed.). Philadelphia: W. B. Saunders.

Kinney, M., Packa, D., & Dunbar, S. (1993). *AACN's clinical reference for critical-care nursing* (3rd ed.). St. Louis: C.V. Mosby.

Kokko, J., & Tannen, R. (1996). *Fluids and electrolytes* (3rd ed.). Philadelphia: W. B. Saunders.

Metheny, N. (1996). *Fluid and electrolyte balance: Nursing considerations* (3rd ed.). Philadelphia: J. B. Lippincott.

Miller, M. (1997). Fluid and electrolyte homeostasis in the elderly: physiologic changes of aging and clinical consequences. *Baillieres Clinical Endocrinology and Metabolism,* 11(2), 367–387.

Narrins, R. (Ed.). (1994). *Maxwell & Kleemans clinical disorders of fluid and electrolyte metabolism* (5th ed.). New York: McGraw-Hill.

North American Nursing Diagnosis Association. Nursing Diagnosis: Definitions and Classifications. The Auth. 1996.

Plante, G. E., Chakir, M., Lehoux, S., & Lortie, M. (1995). Disorders of body fluid balance: A new look into the mechanisms of disease. *Canadian Journal of Cardiology,* 11(9), 788–802.

Porth, C. (1994). *Pathophysiology: Concepts of altered health states* (4th ed.). Philadelphia: J. B. Lippincott.

Rose, B. (1994). *Clinical physiology of acid-base and electrolyte disorders* (4th ed.). New York: McGraw-Hill.

Seaman, S. L. (1995). Renal physiology part II: Fluid and electrolyte regulation. *Neonatal network,* 14(5), 5–11.

Smith, K., & Brain, E. (1991). *Fluids and electrolytes: A conceptual approach* (2nd ed.). New York: Churchill Livingstone.

Szerlip, H., & Goldfarb, S. (1993). *Workshops in fluid and electrolyte disorders.* New York: Churchill Livingstone.

Toto, K. (1994). Endocrine physiology. *Critical Care Nursing Clinics of North America,* December, 647–657.

STUDY QUESTIONS

1. A patient's arterial blood gas (ABG) values are pH 7.34, PaCO₂ 44, HCO₃ 28; the nurse would analyze these findings as indicating:
   a. respiratory acidosis, uncompensated
   b. respiratory acidosis, partially compensated
   c. metabolic acidosis, uncompensated
   d. metabolic acidosis, partially compensated

2. When assessing a patient for respiratory alkalosis, the nurse would *not* expect to observe:
   a. confusion
   b. hypoventilation
   c. cyanosis
   d. syncope

3. Nursing interventions for respiratory alkalosis include:
   a. cupping and clapping
   b. suctioning
   c. using a rebreathing mask
   d. administering oxygen

4. The body's compensation for respiratory alkalosis involves:
   a. decreased excretion of bicarbonate
   b. increased excretion of bicarbonate
   c. increased excretion of hydrogen ions
   d. increased retention of bicarbonate

5. When assessing a patient for metabolic acidosis, the nurse would expect to assess:
   a. carpopedal spasm
   b. tetany
   c. hypokalemia
   d. Kussmaul's respirations

6. Which of the following series of ABG values indicates uncompensated metabolic acidosis?
   a. pH 7.32, PaCO₂ 43, HCO₃ 26
   b. pH 7.32, PaCO₂ 43, HCO₃ 28
   c. pH 7.32, PaCO₂ 32, HCO₃ 20
   d. pH 7.32, PaCO₂ 38, HCO₃ 20

7. The body attempts to compensate for metabolic acidosis by:
   a. increasing the respiratory rate
   b. decreasing the respiratory rate
   c. increasing urinary output
   d. decreasing urinary output

8. Concomitant electrolyte alterations commonly observed in metabolic alkalosis include:
   a. decreased serum potassium and chloride
   b. increased serum potassium and chloride
   c. decreased serum sodium
   d. increased serum potassium and sodium

9. In reviewing the laboratory data for a patient with suspected respiratory acidosis, the nurse is aware that which of the following ABG components would confirm that the problem is, indeed, respiratory and not metabolic?
   a. pH
   b. PaCO₂
   c. HCO₃
   d. none of the above

10. Nursing interventions for a patient in respiratory acidosis with a nursing diagnosis of activity intolerance would include:
    a. suctioning airway to maintain patency
    b. forcing fluids
    c. instituting chest physiotherapy
    d. planning the patient's activities to allow for rest

11. Vomiting or gastric drainage can lead to:
    a. respiratory acidosis
    b. respiratory alkalosis
    c. metabolic acidosis
    d. metabolic alkalosis

12. A patient with respiratory alkalosis is sedated. The nurse knows this intervention is effective when:
    a. The pO₂ is 80%
    b. pH is 7.51
    c. pH is 7.36
    d. CO₂ is 75%

ANSWER KEY

Question	Correct answer	Correct answer rationale	Incorrect answer rationales
1.	b	These ABG values indicate respiratory acidosis, partially compensated.	a. ABG values of pH 7.34, $PaCO_2$ 44, HCO_3 26 indicate respiratory acidosis, uncompensated. c. ABG values of pH 7.34, $PaCO_2$ 38, HCO_3 20 indicate metabolic acidosis, uncompensated. d. ABG values of pH 7.34, $PaCO_2$ 36, HCO_3 20 indicate metabolic acidosis, partially uncompensated.
2.	d	Syncope is observed in respiratory alkalosis.	a, b, and c. These are present in respiratory acidosis.
3.	c	Use of a rebreathing mask allows the patient to increase his $PaCO_2$.	a, b, and d. Cupping and clapping, suctioning, and oxygen administration are appropriate interventions for respiratory acidosis.
4.	b	Respiratory alkalosis involves an excessive amount of base in relation to acid; the body attempts to compensate by increasing base [bicarbonate) excretion.	a, c, and d. These responses do not describe the compensation for respiratory alkalosis.
5.	d	Kussmaul's respirations are a classic sign of metabolic acidosis.	a, b, and c. Carpopedal spasm, tetany, and hypokalemia are symptoms of metabolic alkalosis.
6.	d	ABG values of pH 7.32, $PaCO_2$ 38, HCO_3 20 indicate metabolic acidosis.	a. These ABG values indicate respiratory acidosis, uncompensated. b. These ABG values indicate respiratory acidosis, partially compensated c. These ABG values indicate metabolic acidosis, partially compensated.
7.	a	The body attempts to compensate for metabolic acidosis by increasing the respiratory rate and therefore "blowing off" acid (carbon dioxide).	b, c, and d. These responses do not describe compensation for metabolic acidosis.
8.	a	Decreased serum potassium and serum chloride are found in metabolic alkalosis.	b, c, and d. These electrolyte fluctuations are not associated with metabolic alkalosis.
9.	c	The HCO_3 is normal, indicating that there is no metabolic component.	a and b. Although laboratory findings in respiratory acidosis reveal alterations in pH and $PaCO_2$, the HCO_3 indicates a metabolic component.

Question	Correct answer	Correct answer rationale	Incorrect answer rationales
10.	d	This is the only nursing intervention specifically related to the diagnosis of activity intolerance.	a, b, and c. These nursing interventions may be appropriate for some of the respiratory-related nursing diagnoses.
11.	d	Vomiting or gastric drainage can lead to metabolic alkalosis from loss of gastric juices that are high in hydrogen ion concentration.	a, b, and c. These acid–base disorders are not associated with excessive gastric drainage.
12.	c	This is a normal pH value, indicating that the intervention is effective.	a and d. These choices are not necessarily associated with respiratory alkalosis. b. This is an alkalotic pH..

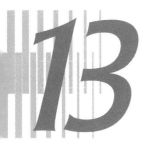

Intravenous (IV) Fluid Replacement Therapy

I.   **Introduction**

A.   Overview of intravenous (IV) fluid replacement therapy

   1.   IV fluid replacement changes the composition of the serum by adding fluids and electrolytes.
2.   Consequently, the nurse must administer IV fluid replacement *with caution* to avoid adverse reactions, which can include:
     a.   Fluid volume excess (FVE)
     b.   Fluid volume deficit (FVD)
     c.   Fluid shifts
     d.   Decreased or increased electrolyte levels

B.   Indications

1.   Replacement of abnormal fluid and electrolyte losses, such as may result from surgery, trauma, burns, or gastrointestinal (GI) bleeding
2.   Maintenance of daily fluid and electrolyte needs (eg, in situations in which

the patient is unable to take in or tolerate oral food and fluids [due to GI disorders], or the patient's status is nothing by mouth)

3. Correction of fluid disorders
4. Correction of electrolyte disorders (in conjunction with other therapies)

II. Types of solutions

A. **Isotonic**
   1. An isotonic solution has the same osmolar concentration, or tonicity, as the plasma.
   2. **This means that the proportion of particles to solution infused is the same as that of the serum; as a result, fluid does not shift across the compartments, and the volume of fluid infused distributes equally across the intracellular and extracellular spaces.**
   3. Isotonic solutions include:
      a. 0.9% sodium chloride (normal saline)
      b. Lactated Ringer's solution

B. **Hypotonic**
   1. Hypotonic solutions contain a lower osmolar concentration than the serum.
   2. **This means that the solution infused is more dilute than the plasma, containing more water than particles.**
   3. **When hypotonic solutions are infused, fluid shifts from the extracellular space to the intracellular space to maintain equilibrium.**
   4. **This eventually leads to swelling or "waterlogging" of the cells, known as water intoxication. (See Chapter 5, Sodium: Normal and Altered Balance, for more information.)**
   5. As the swelling increases, the cells eventually rupture.
   6. Hypotonic solutions include:
      a. 5% dextrose and water (D_5W)
      b. 0.45% sodium chloride (half saline)
      c. 0.33% sodium chloride

C. **Hypertonic**
   1. Hypertonic solutions have a higher concentration of particles in solution compared with the plasma.
   2. **To balance the concentration of fluid and particles across fluid compartments, fluid shifts out of the intracellular space into the extracellular space, causing cellular shrinkage or dehydration.**
   3. **This cellular dehydration causes disturbances in the way cells function.**
   4. In addition, the shift of fluid out of the cells causes the extracellular compartment to expand, which, if excessive, can lead to FVE.
   5. Hypertonic solutions include:
      a. 3% sodium chloride

DISPLAY 13-1
Hyperalimentation

- Hyperalimentation, or total parenteral nutrition, involves the parenteral administration of a hypertonic solition (e.g., dextrose 50% or 70%) that contains all of the necessary dietary requirements (e.g., proteins, carbohydrates, minerals, vitamins).
- The high-glucose solution provides a high-calorie intake and spares protein; in a patient who cannot eat, protein wasting may occur because carbohydrates and fats are burned first.
- Hyperalimentation is administered through a central venous catheter.
- Metabolic complications of hyperalimentation include hyperglycemia or electrolyte disorders if appropriate amounts of elements are not contained in the solution.

        b.   Protein solutions
        c.   Hyperalimentation solutions of 10%, 50%, and 70% dextrose (see Display 13-1)
  6. Table 13-1 describes common isotonic, hypotonic, and hypertonic solutions.

D. Colloids

  1. *Colloids* are fluids that contain solutes of a higher molecular weight (eg, protein); this is in contrast to *crystalloids*, which are electrolyte solutions (eg, D_5W, lactated Ringer's solution, 0.9% normal saline).
  2. Colloid solutions have significant osmotic activity and are hypertonic.

   3. **The presence of colloids in the vascular space pulls fluids from the interstitial and intercellular spaces.**
  4. This osmotic activity makes colloid solutions useful for:
        a.   Mobilizing third-spaced fluids
        b.   Correcting hypotension
        c.   Expanding intravascular volume
        d.   Replenishing protein depletion (such as occurs with liver and renal disease, starvation, GI disease, and multisystem organ failure)
  5. Colloids include:
        a.   Salt pour albumin
        b.   Plasmanate
        c.   Dextran
        d.   Hetastarch (Hespan)
  6. Salt pour albumin contains a highly concentrated solution of albumin in a small volume of fluid.
  7. Plasmanate contains albumin, globulins, and fibrinogen, in a higher fluid volume than salt pour albumin.
  8. Dextran is a highly concentrated glucose solution; it may interfere with blood coagulation.
  9. Hetastarch also interferes with blood coagulation.
 10. All colloids must be used *with extreme caution* because they move fluid from intracellular and interstitial spaces into the intravascular space, risking congestive heart failure and pulmonary edema.

TABLE 13-1
Contents of Selected Water and Electrolyte Solutions with Comments about Their Use

SOLUTION	COMMENTS
5% dextrose in water (D_5W): No electrolytes 50 g of dextrose	Supplies approximately 170 cal/L and free water to aid in renal excretion of solutes Should not be used in excessive volumes in patients with increased ADH activity or to replace fluids in hypovolemic patients
0.9% NaCl (isotonic saline): Na^+ 154 mEq/L Cl^- 154 mEq/L	Isotonic fluid commonly used to expand the extracellular fluid in presence of hypovolemia Because of relatively high chloride content, it can be used to treat mild metabolic alkalosis
0.45% NaCl (½-strength saline): Na^+ 77 mEq/L Cl^- 77 mEq/L	A hypotonic solution that provides Na^+, Cl^-, and free water (Na^+ and Cl^- provided in fluid allow kidneys to select and retain needed amounts) Free water desirable as aid to kidneys in elimination of solutes
0.33% NaCl (1/3-strength saline): Na^+ 56 mEq/L Cl^- 56 mEq/L	A hypotonic solution that provides Na^+, Cl^-, and free water Often used to treat hypernatremia (because this solution contains a small amount of Na^+, it dilutes the plasma sodium while not allowing it to drop too rapidly.)
3% NaCl: Na^+ 513 mEq/L Cl^- 513 mEq/L	Grossly hypertonic solutions used only to treat severe hyponatremia See summary of important nursing considerations in administration
5% NaCl: Na^+ 855 mEq/L Cl^- 855 mEq/L	Dangerous solutions
Lactated Ringer's solution: Na^+ 130 mEq/L K^+ 4 mEq/L Ca^{2+} 3 mEq/L Cl^- 109 mEq/L Lactate (metabolized to bicarbonate) 28 mEq/L	A roughly isotonic solution that contains multiple electrolytes in approximately the same concentrations as found in plasma (Note that this solution is lacking in Mg and PO_4.) Used in the treatment of hypovolemia, burns, and fluid lost as bile or diarrhea Useful in treating mild metabolic acidosis
Sodium lactate solution, 1/6 M: Na^+ 167 mEq/L Cl^- 167 mEq/L	A roughly isotonic solution used to correct severe metabolic acidosis (Lactate is metabolized to bicarbonate in 1–2 hr by the liver.) Not used in patients with liver disease (lactate cannot be converted to bicarbonate in such individuals), also not used in patients with oxygen lack (unable to adequately convert lactate to bicarbonate)
Sodium bicarbonate 5% Na^+ 595 mEq/L Cl^- 595 mEq/L	A very hypertonic solution used to correct severe metabolic acidosis Should be cautiously administered at a slow rate, under careful volume control Should be administered only with extreme caution to salt-retaining patients (e.g., those with cardiac, renal, or liver damage)
Ammonium chloride, 2.14%	Acidifying solution used to correct severe metabolic alkalosis Due to high ammonium content, must be administered cautiously to patients with compromised hepatic function
Potassium chloride, 0.15% K^+ 20 mEq/L Cl^- 20 mEq/L	Premixed potassium chloride solution
Potassium chloride, 0.30% K^+ 40 mEq/L Cl^- 40 mEq/L	Premixed potassium chloride solution

(Source: Metheny, N. M. (1996). Fluid and electrolyte balance (3rd ed.). Philadelphia: Lippincott-Raven, p. 183.)

III. **Replacement with blood products**

A. **Indications**
1. Blood products are required when large volumes of blood or body fluids have been lost.
2. To evaluate a patient's need for blood transfusions, the nurse would assess:
   a. Hemoglobin
   b. Hematocrit
   c. Cardiac output
   d. Swan-Ganz readings (if available)
   e. Vital signs
   f. Urinary output
   g. Skin perfusion
3. Blood transfusions are done only when absolutely necessary, and all blood donors are tested for the presence of human immunodeficiency virus.

B. **Types of blood products**
1. Types of blood products commonly used for transfusions include packed red blood cells (PRBC), fresh frozen plasma (FFP), platelets, and cryoprecipitate (Table 13-2); whole blood is rarely used as a transfusion.
2. *PRBCs:*
   a. Include a large volume of red blood cells (150 mL) in 100 mL of plasma
   b. Elevate hemoglobin levels quickly because they are so concentrated
3. *FFP:*
   a. Contains plasma proteins and clotting factors in a total volume of 200 to 250 mL
   b. Is indicated in patients with large fluid volume losses and in those with coagulation disorders (eg, patients with liver disorders)
   c. Expands the ECF because it is hypertonic
4. *Platelets:*
   a. Are highly concentrated in 50 mL
   b. Are indicated when platelet levels drop below 10,000 mg/dL

TABLE 13-2
Comparison of Blood Products

BLOOD PRODUCT	CONSTITUENTS	VOLUME (mL PER UNIT)
Packed red blood cells	Red blood cells Plasma (100 mL)	250 mL
Fresh frozen plasma	Plasma without red blood cells Plasma proteins Clotting factors (fibrinogen, albumin, and globulins)	200–250 mL
Platelets	Platelets only	50 mL
Cryoprecipitate	Fibrinogen Clotting factor VIII and XIII	10–25 mL

      c.   Are administered as a separate transfusion

5. *Cryoprecipitate:*
    a.   Includes clotting factors and fibrinogen in 10 to 25 mL
    b.   Is indicated when clotting profiles are so high that the patient may bleed to death

IV. Starting an infusion

A. IV equipment
    1.   Alcohol swabs
    2.   Tourniquet
    3.   Angiocatheters
    4.   IV solution
    5.   IV tubing
    6.   IV extension tubing
    7.   Infusion pump (optional)

B. Site selection
    1.   To select an appropriate vein, the nurse must assess the veins of both arms.
    2.   **Veins that are thin, scarred, or in poor condition should be avoided because they will not be able to accommodate the hydrostatic pressure caused by an infusion.**
    3.   Other factors to consider when selecting a vein include:
        a.   Patient comfort and mobility
        b.   Existence of other medical conditions (eg, postmastectomy status or presence of arteriovenous fistulas and grafts); in these conditions, an infusion is contraindicated on the affected side.
        c.   Viscosity and content of the solution and rate of flow; thicker (eg, colloids or blood products) or irritating solutions (eg, potassium chloride) will require larger veins.
    4.   Common sites for IV cannulation include the lower cephalic or basilic veins in the lower forearm and the superficial veins of the hand (Fig. 13-1).
    5.   An IV should not be inserted in the joint (elbow or wrist).
    6.   **Central lines are specialized IV catheters that go into the central circulation:**
        a.   **They may be inserted through the jugular or subclavian veins or through the periphery.**
        b.   **The line passes into the vena cava just above the right atrium.**
        c.   **Because these types of catheters are more invasive, they are not appropriate for short-term use.**

V. Nursing management

A. Initiating therapy
    1.   Ensure that the proper solution is prescribed to meet the patient's needs or that blood products have been properly typed and cross-matched.

    2.   **Ensure that the catheter size is appropriate for the patient and for the vein selected.**

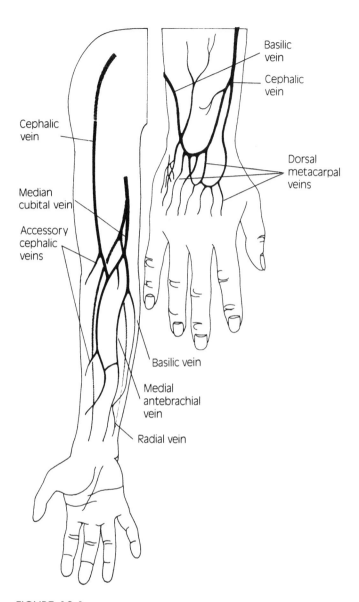

Basilic vein

Cephalic vein

Cephalic vein

Dorsal metacarpal veins

Median cubital vein

Accessory cephalic veins

Basilic vein

Medial antebrachial vein

Radial vein

FIGURE 13-1.
Infusion sites on the ventral and dorsal aspects of the lower arm and hand.

3. **Select a vein that is large enough to accommodate the fluid and that does not restrict mobility.**

4. Maintain asepsis while preparing equipment, preparing the site, and inserting the catheter.

5. Take the patient's temperature before administering blood products.

   6. **Administer blood products with a filter so that no bacteria or small blood clots can pass through to the patient.**
   7. Be aware that different blood products infuse over different times:
     a. PRBC: Infuse over 2 to 4 hours
     b. FFP: Infuse over 1 to 1–12 hours
     c. Platelets: Infuse quickly
     d. Cryoprecipitate: Infuse quickly
   8. See Display 13-2 for issues to consider when instituting IV therapy.

B. Monitoring therapy
   1. Ensure that the IV catheter is secured.
   2. Monitor the infusion site to determine integrity of the vein. Phlebitis or infiltration are two possible complications of intravenous infusion.
   3. Ensure that the appropriate solution or blood product is infusing at all times.
   4. Check that the flow rate remains appropriate.
   5. Monitor for signs of FVE or FVD.
   6. When blood products are used, take and record the patient's temperature during the infusion.
   7. Check hospital protocol to determine how often the dressing and catheter should be changed.
   8. Use aseptic technique when changing an IV dressing.

C. Assessing for adverse reactions
   1. Assess for FVE, which would occur if the patient's heart is unable to accommodate the amount of fluid given; symptoms can include:
     a. Full, bounding pulse
     b. Rales in the lungs
     c. Distended jugular veins
     d. Weight gain
   2. Assess for FVD, which would occur if too little fluid is given and the patient's fluid needs are not met; symptoms can include:

DISPLAY 13-2
Intravenous Replacement Therapy: Questions to Consider

Before the Infusion:
- What is the patient's fluid status (e.g., fluid volume excess or fluid volume deficit)?
- How much fluid can the patient's heart tolerate?
- How much fluid can the patient's kidneys tolerate?
- Does an electrolyte imbalance exist?
- Will the infusion cause a fluid shift?
- Is the solution or blood product appropriate for the patient's present condition?

During the infusion
- Does the solution or blood product being infused still meet the patient's current needs?

After the infusion:
- What effect has the infusion had on the patient?
- Has the treatment objective been achieved?

   a. Poor skin turgor
   b. Dry mucous membranes
   c. Tachycardia
   d. Hypotension
   e. Oliguria
3. Assess for electrolyte imbalances; symptoms can include:
   a. EKG changes
   b. Changes in level of consciousness
   c. Muscle weakness, twitching, or paresthesias
D. Handling complications
   1. IV infusions:
      a. Local and systemic complications may occur as a result of IV therapy (Table 13-3).
      b. Common local complications include phlebitis and infiltration.
      c. Infection is a significant systemic complication that requires discontinuation of the infusion and immediate treatment of the pathogen.
   2. Blood transfusions:
      a. An increase in temperature indicates a possible transfusion reaction and requires immediate discontinuation of the infusion.
      b. Extreme transfusion reactions (eg, anaphylaxis) can be life-threatening (Table 13-4).

TABLE 13-3
Complications Associated with Intravenous Infusions

NAME AND DEFINITION	CAUSES	SIGNS AND SYMPTOMS	NURSING CONSIDERATIONS
Infiltration: The escape of fluid into the subcutaneous tissue	• Dislodged needle • Penetrated vessel wall	Swelling, pallor, coldness, or pain around the infusion site; significant decrease in the flow rate	• Check the infusion site often for symptoms. • Discontinue the infusion if symptoms occur. • Restart the infusion at a different site. • Limit the movement of the extremity with the IV.
Phlebitis: An inflammation of a vein	• Mechanical trauma from needle or catheter • Chemical trauma from solution • Septic (due to contamination)	Local, acute tenderness; redness, warmth, and slight edema of the vein above the insertion site	• Discontinue the infusion immediately. • Apply warm, moist compresses to the affected site. • Avoid further use of the vein. • Restart the infusion in another vein.
Thrombus: A blood clot	• Tissue trauma from needle or catheter	Symptoms similar to phlebitis IV fluid flow may cease if clot obstructs needle	• Stop the infusion immediately. • Apply warm compresses as ordered by the physician.

(continued)

TABLE 13-3
Complications Associated with Intravenous Infusions (*Continued*)

NAME AND DEFINITION	CAUSES	SIGNS AND SYMPTOMS	NURSING CONSIDERATIONS
			• Restart the IV at another site. • *Do not rub or massage the affected area.*
Speed shock: The body's reaction to a substance that is injected into the circulatory system too rapidly	• Too rapid a rate of fluid infusion into circulation	Pounding headache, fainting, rapid pulse rate, apprehension, chills, back pains, and dyspnea	• If symptoms develop, discontinue the infusion immediately. • Report symptoms of speed shock to the physician immediately. • Monitor vital signs if symptoms develop. • Use the proper IV tubing. A microdrip (60 gtt/mL) should be used on all pediatric clients. • Carefully monitor the rate of fluid flow. • Check the rate frequently for accuracy. A time tape is useful for this purpose.
Fluid overload: The condition caused when too large a volume of fluid infuses into the circulatory system	• Too large a volume of fluid infused into circulation	Engorged neck veins, increased blood pressure, and difficulty in breathing (dyspnea)	• If symptoms develop, slow the rate of infusion. • Notify the physician immediately. • Monitor vital signs. • Carefully monitor the rate of fluid flow. • Check the rate frequently for accuracy.
Embolus: A foreign body or air in the circulatory system	• Thrombus dislodges and circulates in the blood • Air enters the vein through the infusion line	Dependent on whether the embolism causes an obstruction or infarction in the circulatory system	• Check the site regularly to identify signs of phlebitis. • Do not allow air to enter the infusion line. • Treat phlebitis with the utmost caution. • Report any sudden pain or breathing difficulty immediately.
Infection: An invasion of pathogenic organisms into the body	• Nonsterile technique used in starting infusion • Improper care of infusion site	Fever; malaise; and pain, swelling, inflammation, or discharge at IV insertion site	• Use scrupulous aseptic technique when starting an infusion. • Change the dressing over the site regularly.

(continued)

TABLE 13-3
Complications Associated with Intravenous Infusions (*Continued*)

NAME AND DEFINITION	CAUSES	SIGNS AND SYMPTOMS	NURSING CONSIDERATIONS
	• Contaminated IV solution		• Change IV tubing every 24 hours if agency policy permits. • Always wash hands before working with the IV.

(Source: Taylor, C. Lillis, C. & LeMone, P. (1997) Fundamentals of Nursing (3rd ed.). Philadelphia: Lippincott-Raven.)

TABLE 13-4
Transfusion Reactions

REACTION	SIGNS AND SYMPTOMS	NURSING ACTIVITY
Allergic reactions: Allergy to transfused blood	Hives, itching Anaphylaxis	• Stop transfusion immediately and keep vein open with normal saline. • Notify physician stat. • Administer antihistamine parenterally as necessary.
Febrile reaction: Fever develops during infusion	Fever and chills Headache Malaise	• Stop transfusion immediately and keep vein open with normal saline. • Notify physician. • Treat symptoms.
Hemolytic transfusion reaction: Incompatibility of blood product	Immediate onset Facial flushing Fever, chills Headache Low back pain Shock	• Stop infusion immediately and keep vein open with normal saline. • Notify physician stat. • Obtain blood samples from site. • Obtain first voided urine. • Treat shock if present. • Send unit, tubing, and filter to lab. • Draw blood sample for serologic testing and send urine specimen to the lab.
Cirulcatory overload: Too much blood administered	Dyspnea Dry cough Pulmonary edema	• Slow or stop infusion. • Monitor vital signs. • Notify physician. • Place in upright position with feet dependent.
Bacterial reaction: Bacteria present in blood	Fever Hypertension Dry, flushed skin Abdominal pain	• Stop infusion immediately. • Obtain culture of client's blood and return blood bag to lab. • Monitor vital signs. • Notify physician. • Administer antibiotics stat.

(Source: Taylor, C., Lillis, C. & LeMone, P. (1993). Fundamentals of Nursing (2nd ed.). Philadelphia: J. B. Lippincott.)

Bibliography

Bullock, B. (1996). *Pathophysiology: Adaptations and alterations in function* (4th ed.). Philadelphia: J. B. Lippincott.

Drummer, C., Gerzer, R., Heer, M., et al. (1992). Effects of an acute saline infusion on fluid and electrolyte metabolism in humans. *American Journal of Physiology,* May, 744–754.

Guyton, A. (1991). *Textbook of medical physiology* (8th ed.). Philadelphia: W. B. Saunders.

Kinney, M., Packa, D., & Dunbar, S. (1993). *AACN's clinical reference for critical-care nursing* (3rd ed.). St. Louis: C.V. Mosby.

Kokko, J., & Tannen, R. (1996). *Fluids and electrolytes* (3rd ed.). Philadelphia: W. B. Saunders.

Metheny, N. (1996). *Fluid and electrolyte balance: Nursing considerations* (3rd ed.). Philadelphia: J. B. Lippincott.

Miller, M. (1997). Fluid and electrolyte homeostasis in the elderly: physiologic changes of aging and clinical consequences. *Baillieres Clinical Endocrinology and Metabolism,* 11(2), 367–387.

Narrins, R. (Ed). (1994). *Maxwell & Kleemans clinical disorders of fluid and electrolyte metabolism* (5th ed.). New York: McGraw-Hill.

North American Nursing Diagnosis Association. Nursing Diagnosis: Definitions and Classifications. The Auth. 1996.

Plante, G. E., Chakir, M., Lehoux, S., & Lortie, M. (1995). Disorders of body fluid balance: A new look into the mechanisms of disease. *Canadian Journal of Cardiology,* 11(9), 788–802.

Porth, C. (1994). *Pathophysiology: Concepts of altered health states* (4th ed.). Philadelphia: J. B. Lippincott.

Rose, B. (1994). *Clinical physiology of acid-base and electrolyte disorders* (4th ed.). New York: McGraw-Hill.

Seaman, S. L. (1995). Renal physiology part II: Fluid and electrolyte regulation. *Neonatal network,* 14(5), 5–11.

Smith, K., & Brain, E. (1991). *Fluids and electrolytes: A conceptual approach* (2nd ed.). New York: Churchill Livingstone.

Szerlip, H., & Goldfarb, S. (1993). *Workshops in fluid and electrolyte disorders.* New York: Churchill Livingstone.

Toto, K. (1994). Endocrine physiology. *Critical Care Nursing Clinics of North America,* December, 647–657.

STUDY QUESTIONS

1. Which of the following solution types is used to replace protein loss occurring secondary to liver disease?
   a. crystalloid
   b. colloids
   c. hypotonic
   d. isotonic

2. Cellular dehydration can result from infusion of:
   a. hypotonic solutions
   b. hypertonic solutions
   c. isotonic solutions
   d. plasmanate

3. Which of the following findings would the nurse *not* expect to assess in a patient with fluid volume excess (FVE)?
   a. bradycardia
   b. bulging neck veins
   c. tachycardia
   d. weight loss

4. Nursing management for a patient receiving hypotonic fluids includes monitoring for which of the following potential complications?
   a. water intoxication
   b. FVE
   c. cellular shrinkage
   d. cell dehydration

5. The nurse would select which one of the following solutions for a patient who is to receive a hypertonic solution?
   a. 0.9% normal saline
   b. 5% dextrose and water
   c. 0.45% normal saline
   d. 3% normal saline

6. When administering a solution with the same osmolar concentration as plasma, the nurse is aware that:
   a. fluid will shift from the extracellular to the interstitial space.
   b. fluid will shift from the intracellular to the interstitial space.
   c. fluid will shift from the plasma to the intracellular space.
   d. no fluid will shift across compartments.

7. When selecting a site for intravenous fluid administration, the nurse would consider all of the following parameters *except:*
   a. body weight
   b. pulse
   c. prescribed infusion
   d. skin turgor

8. Which of the following solutions is a highly concentrated glucose solution that might interfere with coagulation?
   a. Plasmanate
   b. fibrinogen
   c. dextran
   d. salt pour albumin

9. A patient is receiving salt pour albumin every 4 hours. The nurse would monitor the patient for:
   a. renal failure
   b. diabetes
   c. congestive heart failure
   d. Cushing's syndrome

10. A patient will require an IV infusion of Plasmanate, and the nurse will start the infusion. The patient has a history of a right-sided mastectomy. The nurse should take which of the following actions?
    a. Start the IV in a large vein on the patient's left side.
    b. Inform the physician, since a central line will be needed.
    c. Start the IV in a smaller vein on the patient's right side.
    d. Start the IV with a small-gauge cannula on the patient's right side.

ANSWER KEY

Question	Correct answer	Correct answer rationale	Incorrect answer rationales
1.	b	Colloids are hypertonic solutions containing solutes of high molecular weight that pull fluids from the intracellular and interstitial spaces; these solutions are used to replenish protein depletion in liver and renal diseases.	a. Crystalloids are intravenous solutions with solutes of lower molecular weight (eg, 5% dextrose and water and 0.9% normal saline). c and d. These are crystalloids.
2.	b	Hypertonic solutions produce a fluid shift out of the intracellular space into the extracellular space, causing cellular shrinkage or dehydration.	a. Hypotonic solutions produce cellular swelling. c. Isotonic solutions produce no fluid shifts d. Plasmanate is a colloid.
3.	b	Bulging neck veins are a characteristic finding of FVE.	a, c, and d. Bradycardia is not a necessary finding in FVE. Tachycardia and weight loss are more commonly associated with FVD.
4.	a	When hypotonic fluids are infused, fluid shifts from the extracellular to the intracellular space; eventually, this leads to swelling and water intoxication.	a, c, and d. FVE, cellular shrinkage, and cell dehydration are potential complications of hypertonic fluid administration.
5.	d	3% saline is a hypertonic solution; that is, it contains a higher concentration of particles in solution than plasma.	a. 0.9% normal saline is isotonic. b and c. 5% dextrose and water and 0.45% normal saline are hypotonic.
6.	d	Because isotonic solutions contain the same osmolar concentration or tonicity of plasma, administration of isotonic solutions results in no fluid shifting across compartments.	a, b, and c. These fluid shifts are not consistent with the situation described.
7.	c	When selecting a site for IV infusion, the nurse must consider the prescribed solution (eg, thicker solutions will require larger bore veins), and patient mobility (eg, avoid a site over a joint).	a, b, and d. Body weight, skin turgor, and pulse are valuable parameters to assess in terms of fluid status. They are not significant to to site selection
8.	c	Dextran is a highly concentrated glucose solution that may interfere with coagulation.	a. Plasmanate contains albumin, globulins and fibrinogen. b. Fibrinogen is a component of plasmanate. d. Salt pour albumin contains a highly concentrated solution of albumin.

Question	Correct answer	Correct answer rationale	Incorrect answer rationales
9.	c	Salt pour albumin is a colloid, which is known to shift fluid from the intracellular and interstitial spaces into the intravascular space. This shift places the patient at risk for congestive heart failure or pulmonary edema.	a, b, and d. These are not related to the risks of colloid use.
10.	a	The existence of other medical conditions is considered as part of IV site selection. A patient who has had a mastectomy should not have an infusion on the affected side.	b. There is no basis for this action. c and d. Thicker or irritating solutions require larger veins.

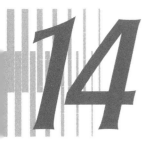

14 Assessing Fluid, Electrolyte, and Acid–Base Balance

I.   Introduction

  A.   **Assessment goals**

     1.   To assess a patient's potential or actual alterations in fluid, electrolyte, or acid–base balance, the nurse must conduct a thorough clinical assessment.

     2.   Specific assessment goals include:
        a.   Ascertaining the body's capability to regulate fluid volume and body fluid composition
        b.   Evaluating the body's effectiveness in maintaining normal acid–base balance
        c.   Delineating specific aspects of fluid, electrolyte, or acid–base imbalance
        d.   Identifying the severity of the fluid, electrolyte, or acid–base imbalance
        e.   Determining the possible causes of abnormalities
        f.   Incorporating appropriate nursing interventions into the patient's care plan

  B.   **Assessment parameters**

     1.   As suggested by Metheny (1996), the nurse must consider particular parameters when assessing a patient for fluid, electrolyte, and acid–base imbalances.

     2.   These key parameters include:
        a.   **Intake and output**
        b.   **Urine volume and concentration**
        c.   **Skin signs (eg, turgor, temperature, and moisture)**
        d.   **Weight**
        e.   **Subjective complaints of thirst**
        f.   **Objective measures of fluid loss, such as tearing or salivation**
        g.   **Edema**

      h. **Cardiovascular signs (eg, pulse, blood pressure, central venous pressure, and respirations)**

      i. **Neuromuscular signs**

II. Intake and output

A. **Normal findings**

1. When measuring a patient's *intake,* the nurse should include:
   a. All fluids taken in by mouth or by intravenous, nasogastric, or nasointestinal administration
   b. Foods high in fluid content (eg, gelatin, ice cream)
   c. Electrolytes and nonelectrolytes ingested or administered
2. When measuring a patient's *output,* the nurse should include:
   a. Urine
   b. Fluid and electrolyte losses through the skin and gastrointestinal (GI) and respiratory tracts
   c. Drainage from fistulas or body cavities
   d. Fluids that have shifted into third spaces
3. Because of the ability to concentrate fluids, normal kidneys maintain electrolyte and acid–base balance even when urine output is decreased to approximately 500 mL/d; as a person ages, urine-concentrating capability decreases.
4. **Normal intake should approximately match urinary output plus extrarenal losses.**

B. **Altered findings**

1. Decreased urine output and symptoms of dehydration
2. Edema formation
3. Altered amount of fluid and electrolyte excretion through the kidneys
4. Oliguria or anuria
5. Positive balance (occurs when intake exceeds output, including insensible loss)
6. Negative balance (occurs when output exceeds intake)

C. **Possible causes of alterations**

1. Excessive free water intake
2. Inadequate intake
3. Renal disease, such as:
   a. Acute tubular necrosis
   b. Acute renal failure
   c. Chronic renal failure
   d. Renal salt wasting
4. Cardiovascular disease, such as:
   a. Congestive heart failure (CHF)
   b. Cardiomyopathy
5. Iatrogenic administration of fluids
6. Excessive nasogastric drainage
7. Endocrine disorders (eg, syndrome of inappropriate antidiuretic hormone and diabetes insipidus)

8. Frank blood or volume loss
9. Third-space fluid shifting secondary to hepatic disease or due to fluid redistribution as found in burn injuries

 10. **Causes of excessive extrarenal fluid losses can include:**
  a. **Fever: Elevations in temperature result in increased fluid loss through the skin.**
  b. **Hyperventilation: A ventilation rate that exceeds the body's metabolic needs results in increased insensible loss through the respiratory tract.**
  c. **Ambient temperature: Hot, dry climates increase integumentary losses by evaporative processes.**
  d. **GI losses: Diarrhea, vomiting, nasogastric drainage, and fistula drainage increase the amount of fluid and electrolyte losses.**
  e. **Distributive loss: Third-space shifting into pleural or peritoneal cavities, diffuse capillary leakage (as in liver or renal disease), and evaporative and transudative losses (as in a significant burn injury) increase fluid and electrolyte loss.**

III.   Urine volume

A.   Normal findings
  1. In a patient with functioning kidneys, normal urine output is approximately 600 mL/d.
  2. Urine output will increase depending on the patient's intake and the amount of insensible loss.
  3. Baseline urine output in most clinical settings is approximately 30 mL/h.

B.   Altered findings
  1. Low urine volume
  2. High urine volume

C.   Possible causes of alterations
  1. Acute or chronic renal failure
  2. Fluid volume deficit (FVD) or fluid volume excess (FVE) due to any cause
  3. Redistributive conditions (eg, pancreatitis, burn injury, ascites, CHF)
  4. Diuresis

IV.   Urine concentration

A.   Normal findings
  1. The kidneys can reabsorb filtered water in relation to the degree of systemic hydration. The amount of fluid reabsorbed depends on the patient's hydration status and the amount of circulating ADH.
  2. The measure of urine concentration is the *specific gravity*. Specific gravity depends not only on hydration status, but also on the existence of solutes (eg, protein, glucose).
  3. A normal specific gravity is between 1.003 and 1.035.

    4. A more specific measure of concentration is *urine osmolality,* which is a measure of the total number of particles in solution, independent of the size and molecular weight of those particles.

    5. A normal urine osmolality depends on a number of clinical parameters, but an acceptable range is 50 mOsm/kg to 1200 mOsm/kg.

B. Altered findings

    1. Elevated specific gravity and urine osmolality

    2. Low specific gravity and urine osmolality

C. Possible causes of alterations

    1. Elevated findings may be associated with:

        a. Hypernatremia

        b. FVD

        c. Clearance of high-molecular-weight solutes (eg, contrast media)

    2. Low findings may be associated with:

        a. Hyponatremia

        b. FVE

        c. Renal failure

        d. FVD

V. Skin turgor

A. Normal findings

    1. Skin turgor indicates a patient's hydration status.

    2. Skin with normal turgor moves easily when lifted and returns rapidly to its previous position.

    3. Elderly patients tend to have less skin elasticity, so pinched skin returns more slowly to its normal position when released.

B. Altered findings

    1. Poor skin turgor (eg, skin that remains elevated when lifted or "tents" or that takes a prolonged time to return to its normal position when released)

    2. In edematous conditions, skin turgor that may be within normal limits but with fragile skin that is prone to breakdown

C. Possible causes of alterations

    1. FVD

    2. Peripheral edema

VI. Tongue turgor and mucous membrane moisture

A. Normal findings

    1. Normally the tongue is covered with papillae on the dorsum and is smooth underneath.

    2. In a patient with normal hydration, the tongue is moist and has no evidence of fissures (cracks in the surface).

    3. The oral cavity also is moist, and membranes (including the lips) are smooth and intact.

B. Altered findings
   1. Dry tongue with visible fissures or furrows
   2. Dry membranes
   3. Viscous mucus
   4. Cracked and chapped lips
C. Possible causes of alterations
   1. FVD due to conditions such as:
      a. Frank blood loss
      b. GI losses
      c. Excessive diuretic therapy
   2. Hypernatremia due to conditions such as:
      a. Primary hyperaldosteronism
      b. Diabetes insipidus
      c. Burns

VII. Body weight

A. Normal findings
   1. Total body weight (TBW) depends on the patient's height, sex, and bone structure.
   2. **Fluid status also plays a role in the determination of TBW. ECF represents approximately 20% of total body weight; ICF, approximately 40%.**
   3. **One liter of fluid is approximately equivalent to 1 kg (2.2 lb) of TBW; therefore, the loss or gain of 1 kg of TBW indicates approximately 1 L of combined ECF and ICF fluid loss or gain.**
   4. In a healthy adult, TBW should remain relatively unchanged.
   5. **In a patient with third-space fluid shifting, weight gain may occur despite FVD in the intravascular space.**
B. Altered findings
   1. Rapid weight loss, ranging from 2% to 8% of TBW
   2. Rapid weight gain, ranging from 2% to 8% of TBW
C. Possible causes of alterations
   1. Rapid weight loss is associated with FVD and hypernatremia.
   2. Rapid weight gain is associated with FVE, particularly conditions in which there is significant edema.

VIII. Thirst

A. Normal findings
   1. The thirst center is located in the hypothalamus.
   2. As fluid is lost, osmoreceptors shrink to stimulate thirst and increase oral intake.
   3. As hydration status stabilizes, the water content of the osmoreceptors increases, and the thirst response is no longer experienced.

B. **Altered findings**
   1. Increased oral intake due to the thirst response, despite normal hydration status
   2. Poor oral intake despite subjective feelings of thirst
C. **Possible causes of alterations**
   1. Neurologic disorders (eg, head trauma, malignancy, or vascular insult) have been known to cause hypothalamic injury, resulting in deficits in the thirst experience.
   2. Psychogenic polydypsia is a psychologic disease that results in increased fluid intake despite normal hydration status.
   3. Neuromuscular disease or coma result in the inability to take in fluids despite subjective feelings of thirst.

IX. Tearing and salivation

A. **Normal findings**
   1. Tears are produced for the purpose of lubricating the eyes and thus protecting them from abrasions.
   2. Salivation is stimulated by smells, thoughts, or the actual presence of food; its purpose is to lubricate food to facilitate movement into the GI tract.
B. **Altered findings**
   1. Decreased tearing
   2. Decreased salivation
C. **Possible causes of alterations: Causes are the same as for alterations in tongue turgor and mucous membrane moisture (see Section VI.C).**

X. Skin and body temperature

A. **Normal findings**
   1. Normal skin is warm and dry; skin color varies depending on perfusion, but generally it manifests with good turgor and appearance.
   2. Body temperature is approximately 98.6°F or 37°C; variations occur depending on the method of testing and individual idiosyncrasies.
B. **Altered findings**
   1. Elevated skin and body temperature (occur as perspiration decreases and the body is less efficient in maintaining normo-thermia)
   2. Dry, flaky skin
C. **Possible causes of alterations: Causes are the same as for alterations in tongue turgor and mucous membrane moisture (see Section VI.C).**

XI. Edema

A. **Normal findings**
   1. A normal hydration status is not associated with edema.
   2. Skin is normally pliant with good elasticity, but no swelling is present.

B. **Altered findings**
1. Edema (deposition of fluid in the interstitial tissue)
2. Pitting edema (severe interstitial fluid accumulation resulting in the tissue's inability to return to normal configuration after pressure is applied)

 3. **Pulmonary edema (fluid accumulation in the interstitial space. This is life-threatening and develops when the heart can not circulate the fluid volume throughout the body).**

C. **Possible causes of alterations**
1. Peripheral dependent edema is caused by FVE.
2. Edema also can result from vascular abnormalities and systemic conditions (eg, CHF).

XII.   Pulse

A. **Normal findings**
1. The normal pulse is strong and regular.
2. Heart rate is between 60 and 100 beats/min.

B. **Altered findings**
1. Bounding pulse
2. Weak and thready pulse
3. Bradycardia (< 60 beats/min)
4. Tachycardia (> 100 beats/min)

C. **Possible causes of alterations**
1. A bounding pulse is associated with FVE.
2. A weak, thready pulse is associated with impending cardiovascular collapse; causes of cardiovascular collapse include:
   a. Severe FVD
   b. Hyperkalemia
   c. Hypocalcemia
   d. Hyperphosphatemia
3. Bradycardia is associated with hypokalemia and hypermagnesemia.
4. Tachycardia is associated with FVD (it occurs as a compensatory sympathetic nervous system response), respiratory acidosis, and hypernatremia.
5. **Pulse rate irregularities caused by dysrhythmias are associated with metabolic acidosis, metabolic alkalosis, respiratory alkalosis, hypophosphatemia, and hypercalcemia.**

XIII.   Respiration

A. **Normal findings**
1. Normal respiratory rate is between 12 and 20 breaths per minute.
2. Normal respiratory pattern is regular with bilateral chest expansion.
3. Lung sounds are clear to auscultation.

B. **Altered findings**
1. Altered respiratory patterns, including:

      a. Hyperventilation
      b. Hypoventilation
      c. Kussmaul's breathing
   2. Abnormal breaths sounds, such as crackles on auscultation
   3. Increased work of breathing, including dyspnea and dyspnea on exertion
C. Possible causes of alterations
   1. Hyperventilation is associated with hyperchloremia and respiratory alkalosis.
   2. Hypoventilation is associated with metabolic alkalosis, respiratory acidosis, hypokalemia, and hypermagnesemia.
   3. Kussmaul's breathing is associated with metabolic acidosis.
   4. Laryngeal stridor is associated with hypocalcemia and hyperphosphatemia.

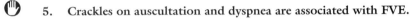   **5. Crackles on auscultation and dyspnea are associated with FVE.**

XIV. Blood pressure

A. Normal findings
   1. Blood pressure is considered within normal ranges if systolic does not exceed 140 mm Hg and diastolic does not exceed 90 mm Hg.
   2. The lower range of acceptable blood pressure includes a systolic of 80 mm Hg and a diastolic of 50 mm Hg.
B. Altered findings
   1. Hypertension (< 140/90 mm Hg)
   2. Hypotension (> 80/50 mm Hg)
   3. Postural hypotension (drop in systolic pressure due to orthostatic changes)
C. Possible causes of alterations
   1. Hypertension is associated with FVE and hypomagnesemia.
   2. Hypotension is associated with FVD, metabolic acidosis, respiratory alkalosis, and hypermagnesemia.
   3. Postural hypotension may be seen in FVD.

XV. Neck veins and central venous pressure (CVP)

A. Normal findings
   1. Venous pressure can be calculated by observing the external jugular veins; visualizing pulsations with measurement to the sternal angle affords an estimate of venous pressure.

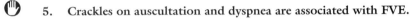   **2. Normal venous pressure is 3 to 4 cm above the sternal angle.**
   3. CVP may be measured directly using a catheter in the vena cava.
   4. Normal CVP reading ranges from 5 to 19 cm of water or 6 to 12 mm Hg.
B. Altered findings
   1. Flat or distended neck veins
   2. Elevated or below-normal CVP
C. Possible causes of alterations
   1. Neck vein distension and elevated CVP readings are associated with FVE.
   2. Flattened neck veins and low CVP readings are associated with FVD.

XVI. Neuromuscular irritability

A. **Normal findings:** Intact neurologic function (eg, normal cognitive, motor, and sensory findings)

B. **Altered findings**

   1. **Cognitive changes, ranging from mild alterations (eg, restlessness, irritability, and decreased mentation) to severe alterations (eg, disorientation and coma)**

   2. Motor dysfunction (eg, fatigue or muscle weakness); may be associated with lack of coordination or decreased reflex response

   3. Severe neuromuscular changes, such as tetany and carpopedal spasms associated with Chvostek's and Trousseau's signs (Fig. 14-1)

   4. Lack of coordination, such as is seen with vertigo, ataxia, and syncope

   5. Sensory changes, including paresthesias, cramping, tetany, and Chvostek's and Trousseau's signs

   6. Severe alterations (eg, seizures and psychoses)

C. **Possible causes of alterations**

   1. Cognitive changes have been associated with:

   a. FVD

   b. Acid–base imbalances

   c. Hypercalcemia

   d. Hypokalemia or hyperkalemia

   e. Hyponatremia or hypernatremia

   f. Hypochloremia or hyperchloremia

   g. Hypomagnesemia or hypermagnesemia

   h. Hypophosphatemia or hyperphosphatemia

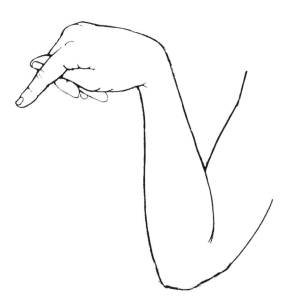

FIGURE 14-1.
Trousseau's sign. Carpopedal spasm with hypocalcemia.

    2. Neuromuscular alterations, such as weakness and tremors are associated with:

        a. Acid–base imbalances

        b. Alterations in potassium, calcium, sodium, magnesium, and chloride balance

    3. Tetany and hyperreflexia are associated with:

        a. Respiratory alkalosis

        b. Hypocalcemia

        c. Hypochloremia

        d. Hypomagnesemia

        e. Hyponatremia

        f. Hyperphosphatemia

    4. Weakness and hyporeflexia are associated with:

        a. Hypokalemia

        b. Hypophosphatemia

        c. Hypercalcemia

        d. Hypermagnesemia

    5. Sensory abnormalities, such as paresthesias, are associated with:

        a. Hypophosphatemia and hyperphosphatemia

        b. Hypomagnesemia

        c. Hyperkalemia

        d. Respiratory alkalosis

XVII. Nursing diagnoses

A. Overview of nursing diagnoses

    1. Nursing diagnoses are conclusions derived from assessment findings; data from the patient history and examination are collected, analyzed, and synthesized. The result of that analysis is a nursing diagnosis.

    2. Accurate nursing diagnosis depends on accurate assessment; an assessment that does not include all necessary parameters will yield inaccurate data, which then yield an incorrect diagnosis.

    3. Nursing diagnoses affect implementation; incorrect diagnoses yield incorrect interventions, which result in poor patient outcomes.

    4. Diagnosing fluid, electrolyte, and acid–base imbalances requires a knowledge of pathophysiology, pharmacology, and fluid therapies and the ability to think critically:

        a. Knowledge of pathophysiology requires an understanding of how a particular disorder affects fluid, electrolyte, and acid–base balance in each patient.

        b. Knowledge of pharmacology requires understanding how various drugs cause increases or decreases in fluid excretion or result in fluid and electrolyte shifts.

        c. Knowledge of fluid therapies requires an understanding of how parenteral therapies change the composition of body fluids and affect electrolyte status.

        d. Critical thinking allows the nurse to correctly analyze patient information and formulate an accurate nursing diagnosis.

5. Nursing diagnoses for fluid, electrolyte, and acid–base imbalances affect all body systems.

B.   Potential nursing diagnoses for fluid, electrolyte, and acid–base imbalances
1. Activity Intolerance
2. Ineffective Airway Clearance
3. Anxiety
4. High Risk for Altered Body Temperature
5. Ineffective Breathing Pattern
6. Decreased Cardiac Output
7. Constipation
8. Diarrhea
9. Fatigue
10. Fluid Volume Deficit
11. Fluid Volume Excess
12. Impaired Gas Exchange
13. Altered Health Maintenance
14. Hyperthermia
15. Hypothermia
16. Altered Nutrition: Less than Body Requirements
17. Altered Oral Mucous Membranes
18. Pain
19. Impaired Skin Integrity
20. Impaired Tissue Perfusion
21. Urinary Elimination

Bibliography

Bullock, B. (1996). *Pathophysiology: Adaptations and alterations in function* (4th ed.). Philadelphia: J. B. Lippincott.

Drummer, C., Gerzer, R., Heer, M., et al. (1992). Effects of an acute saline infusion on fluid and electrolyte metabolism in humans. *American Journal of Physiology,* May, 744–754.

Guyton, A. (1991). *Textbook of medical physiology* (8th ed.). Philadelphia: W. B. Saunders.

Kinney, M., Packa, D., & Dunbar, S. (1993). *AACN's clinical reference for critical-care nursing* (3rd ed.). St. Louis: C.V. Mosby.

Kokko, J., & Tannen, R. (1996). *Fluids and electrolytes* (3rd ed.). Philadelphia: W. B. Saunders.

Metheny, N. (1996). *Fluid and electrolyte balance: Nursing considerations* (3rd ed.). Philadelphia: J. B. Lippincott.

Miller, M. (1997). Fluid and electrolyte homeostasis in the elderly: physiologic changes of aging and clinical consequences. *Baillieres Clinical Endocrinology and Metabolism,* 11(2), 367–387.

Narrins, R. (Ed). (1994). *Maxwell & Kleemans clinical disorders of fluid and electrolyte metabolism* (5th ed.). New York: McGraw-Hill.

North American Nursing Diagnosis Association. Nursing Diagnosis: Definitions and Classifications. The Auth. 1996.

Plante, G. E., Chakir, M., Lehoux, S., & Lortie, M. (1995). Disorders of body fluid balance: A new look into the mechanisms of disease. *Canadian Journal of Cardiology,* 11(9), 788–802.

Porth, C. (1994). *Pathophysiology: Concepts of altered health states* (4th ed.). Philadelphia: J. B. Lippincott.

Rose, B. (1994). *Clinical physiology of acid-base and electrolyte disorders* (4th ed.). New York: McGraw-Hill.

Seaman, S. L. (1995). Renal physiology part II: Fluid and electrolyte regulation. *Neonatal network,* 14(5), 5–11.

Smith, K., & Brain, E. (1991). *Fluids and electrolytes: A conceptual approach* (2nd ed.). New York: Churchill Livingstone.

Szerlip, H., & Goldfarb, S. (1993). *Workshops in fluid and electrolyte disorders.* New York: Churchill Livingstone.

Toto, K. (1994). Endocrine physiology. *Critical Care Nursing Clinics of North America,* December, 647–657.

STUDY QUESTIONS

1. The normal kidney maintains electrolyte and acid–base balance even when urine output is reduced to:
   a. 100 mL/day
   b. 10 mL/hour
   c. 500 mL/day
   d. 1000 mL/day

2. Which of the following findings would the nurse expect to assess in a patient with extrarenal fluid loss?
   a. hypothermia
   b. hypoventilation
   c. diarrhea
   d. distributive gain

3. Which of the following parameters provides information on urine concentration by measuring the total number of particles in solution?
   a. specific gravity
   b. urine osmolarity
   c. urine output
   d. BUN

4. Tachycardia is associated with fluid volume:
   a. deficits as a compensatory sympathetic nervous system response
   b. deficits related to hyponatremia
   c. excesses as a compensatory sympathetic nervous system response
   d. excesses related to fluid overload

5. A patient with chronic renal failure asks the nurse why his fluid intake is restricted. The nurse's best response would be:
   a. "Since your urine output is diminished, you can only ingest the amount you excrete."
   b. "Excessive free water intake will contribute to edema, because renal clearance is a concern."
   c. "Decreasing your oral intake will allow your kidneys to rest and heal."

   d. "Fluids are restricted because of your medication therapy."

6. In a patient with fluid volume excess (FVE), the neck veins appear to be:
   a. distended
   b. flattened
   c. retracted
   d. normal

7. During an examination, a patient exhibits hyperreflexia. The nurse knows that this is associated with:
   a. hypercalcemia
   b. hypermagnesemia
   c. respiratory acidosis
   d. hypocalcemia

8. When assessing a patient for fluid and electrolyte abnormalities, the nurse is aware that hypokalemia may cause:
   a. hyperreflexia
   b. paresthesia
   c. tetany
   d. hyporeflexia

9. When caring for a patient at risk for fluid overload the nurse notices that overnight he gained 6 pounds. The nurse interprets this as:
   a. a 3-L fluid gain
   b. impending renal failure
   c. excessive diuresis
   d. a 6-L fluid gain

10. A nurse is caring for a patient with major burns. During assessment all signs of dehydration are present, yet the intravenous intake matches urinary output. The nurse knows that dehydration occurred through:
    a. the stool
    b. surgical sites
    c. the skin
    d. vomiting

ANSWER KEY

Question	Correct answer	Correct answer rationale	Incorrect answer rationales
1.	c	Because of its ability to concentrate fluids, the normal kidney can maintain electrolyte and acid–base balance even when urine output is reduced to 500 mL/day.	a, b, and d. These responses are incorrect.
2.	c	Extrarenal fluid loss refers to fluid loss that occurs in sites other than the kidney.	a and b. Neither hypothermia nor hypoventilation cause fluid loss. d. This response is incorrect. It refers to a gain rather than a loss.
3.	b	Urine osmolarity is a measure of the total number of particles in solution, independent of size or weight.	a. Specific gravity measures urine concentration but is dependent on the existence of solutes. c. Urine output does not provide information on urine concentration. d. BUN is a blood test.
4.	a	Tachycardia is associated with fluid volume deficits as a compensatory sympathetic nervous system response.	b, c, and d. These responses are incorrect.
5.	b	In a patient with impaired renal clearance, excessive fluid intake can contribute to edema.	a, c, and d. These responses are incorrect.
6.	a	Neck veins are distended in FVE.	b. Flattened neck veins occur in FVD. c. There is no such entity as retracted neck veins. d. Normal neck veins exist when normal fluid balance is present.
7.	d	Hyperreflexia is associated with hypocalcemia.	a. This response is incorrect. b and c. Hypomagnesemia and respiratory alkalosis are associated with hyperreflexia.
8.	d	Hyporeflexia and weakness are associated with hypokalemia.	a and c. Tetany and hyperreflexia not associated with fluctuating potassium levels. b. Paresthesias are associated with hyperkalemia.
9.	a	A sudden gain of this amount points to fluid overload. One liter of fluid is approximately 2 pounds.	b. Inadequate urinary output from renal failure can cause fluid gain, but renal failure is not necessarily the cause. Letter a is the best choice.

Question	Correct answer	Correct answer rationale	Incorrect answer rationales
			c. Excessive diuresis will result in fluid and subsequent weight loss. d. Six liters will result in a 12-pound fluid gain.
10.	c	Fluid lost through the skin can not be measured. In the case of a burn patient, fluid loss can be high volume.	a, b, and d. Large amounts of fluids can be lost through this route, but the situation does not indicate that these choices are as probable as letter c.

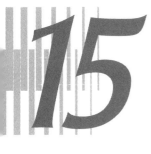

Disorders Associated With High Risk for Fluid, Electrolyte, and Acid–Base Imbalances

I. Introduction

A. Overview of imbalances
   1. Fluid and electrolyte deficiencies tend to be caused by conditions associated with:
      a. Decreased intake
      b. Excessive elimination
   2. Fluid and electrolyte excesses tend to be caused by conditions associated with:
      a. Excessive intake
      b. Decreased elimination
   3. Acid–base imbalances may be caused by metabolic conditions that affect regulatory mechanisms.
   4. Abnormal routes of fluid and electrolyte intake or output can lead to fluid and electrolyte alteration of any type.

B. Types of disorders associated with imbalances
   1. Endocrine disorders in which protein, carbohydrate, or fat metabolism is altered, such as in:
      a. Diabetes insipidus
      b. Syndrome of inappropriate antidiuretic hormone (SIADH)
      c. Diabetic ketoacidosis (DKA)
      d. Hyperglycemic hyperosmolar nonketotic coma (HHNC)
      e. Pancreatitis
   2. Renal disorders in which the buffer systems are inadequate or not functioning
   3. Gastrointestinal (GI) fluid losses due to altered metabolism or elimination
   4. Respiratory disorders
   5. Disorders of decreased cardiac output
   6. Burns
   7. Cirrhosis
   8. Surgery
   9. Malignant disorders

II. Diabetes insipidus (DI)

A. Description and etiology
   1. DI is caused by inadequate secretion of antidiuretic hormone (ADH) from the pituitary gland; this may result from:

    a.   Head trauma
    b.   Cerebral ischemia due to a cerebrovascular accident (CVA)
    c.   Pituitary or brain surgery
    d.   Endocrine disorders

  2. ADH insufficiency reduces the amount of water eliminated in the kidney tubules, increasing urine volume and decreasing extracellular fluid (ECF) volume.

B. **Pathophysiologic processes and clinical manifestations**

  1. As a result of damage to the hypothalamus, the stalk, or the pituitary gland, insufficient amounts of ADH are released.

  2. Lack of ADH allows excessive renal excretion of water, with liters being excreted each hour.

  3. This excessive diuresis results in extracellular fluid volume deficit, which causes hypotension.

  4. Because water is excreted in excess of sodium, hypernatremia occurs.

C. **Overview of nursing interventions**

  1. Administer replacement fluids as prescribed. Replacement fluids should be determined based on the quantity and constituents of fluids lost.

  2. Monitor for hypotension and cardiovascular collapse.

  3. Monitor electrolyte levels.

  4. Monitor intake and output closely.

  5. Administer Vasopressin as prescribed. The type and amount varies with the type and cause of diabetes insipidus present.

III. Syndrome of inappropriate antidiuretic hormone (SIADH)

A. **Description**

  1. SIADH involves continuous pituitary secretion of ADH when plasma osmolarity is low.

  2. This hormonal excess increases the amount of water absorbed by the kidney tubules, decreasing urine volume and resulting in extracellular fluid volume excess (FVE).

B. **Etiology**

  1. Head trauma

  2. Cerebral ischemia due to CVA

  3. Endocrine disorders (eg, hyperpituitarism)

  4. Pulmonary tumors in which the tumor secretes a chemical similar to ADH

  5. Medications such as Dilantin

  6. Brain surgery in which cerebral edema affects hormonal secretion

C. **Pathophysiologic processes and clinical manifestations**

  1. As a result of damage to either the hypothalamic messenger–releasing process or the pituitary gland, excessive amounts of ADH are secreted.

  2. This excess is continuous and unregulated by the usual feedback mechanism.

  3. ADH acts on the distal tubules to reabsorb water; excessive ADH secretion causes excessive water retention, diluting the ECF.

  4. This water retention causes osmolality to drop as particles are diluted, lowering serum osmolality and elevating urine osmolality.

5.   Excessive water retention also increases intravascular volume and blood pressure, inhibiting secretion of renin and aldosterone.

   6.   Aldosterone inhibition reduces sodium absorption, causing hyponatremia through sodium loss. Excessive water retention dilutes sodium, also causing hyponatremia.

   7.   The resulting hyponatremia is profound and life-threatening.

D.   Overview of nursing interventions

1.   Measure and record carefully daily intake and output and weight.
2.   Restrict water intake.
3.   Monitor vital signs frequently.
4.   Monitor serum sodium concentration closely because the cells can become waterlogged, altering the patient's sensorium.
5.   Administer hypertonic saline as ordered if hyponatremia is severe:
    a.   Give hypertonic saline *with caution* because a rapid shift of water from the ICF to ECF can result in congestive heart failure (CHF).
    b.   Administer Lasix with the hypertonic saline as ordered to eliminate excess water shifting into the ECF.

IV.   Diabetic Ketoacidosis (DKA)

A.   Description

1.   DKA is a condition characterized by acute insulin deficiency, resulting in metabolic acidosis due to the presence of ketone bodies (which are produced during fat metabolism).
2.   It commonly occurs in patients with undiagnosed diabetes.

B.   Etiology

1.   Insufficient insulin secretion
2.   Inadequate insulin intake (possibly due to the patient's failure to take insulin as prescribed)
3.   Stressful situations (eg, surgery, infection, emotional stress, trauma) in which steroid hormones are secreted; these hormones act as antagonists to insulin, causing glucose levels to rise.

C.   Pathophysiologic processes and clinical manifestations

1.   As glucose levels rise, hyperglycemia occurs as a lack of insulin prevents use of glucose, the body's primary energy source.
2.   As a result, the body burns fat, its secondary energy source.
3.   Fat metabolism yields ketone bodies as an acid end-product, resulting in metabolic acidosis.
4.   The respiratory system tries to compensate for the increased acids through deep, rapid breathing known as Kussmaul's respirations.
5.   The body tries to eliminate the excess acids by increasing acid excretion, causing ketonuria; ketones also are present in the serum.
6.   The large amount of glucose present in the serum causes hyperosmolality, which produces osmotic diuresis (because glucose tends to attract water); osmotic diuresis causes fluid and electrolyte losses and contributes to hyponatremia.

7. As fluid is eliminated from the intravascular space through the urine, dehydration may result and electrolyte shifts may occur.
8. Hypokalemia occurs as osmotic diuresis promotes potassium excretion and acidemia shifts potassium out of the cells.
9. In response to fluid loss, aldosterone is secreted, causing sodium reabsorption and potassium elimination and further exacerbation of hypokalemia.
10. In response to hyperglycemia, potassium moves from the ECF to the ICF. There are then several mechanisms at work that will cause hypokalemia.

D. **Overview of nursing interventions**
1. Administer regular insulin to decrease serum glucose as ordered; monitor serum glucose levels to avoid overcorrection and hypoglycemia.
2. Administer bicarbonate as ordered if acidosis is severe.

 3. **Monitor serum potassium as potassium moves from the ICF to the ECF during correction of acidosis.**
4. Rehydrate patient as ordered with 0.9% sodium chloride or lactated Ringer's solution; be aware that replacement may need to be rapid (eg, as much as 1 L/h).
6. Assess fluid volume status, and maintain blood pressure.
7. Measure and record carefully intake and output; insert a Foley catheter to obtain hourly measurements.
8. Monitor hemodynamic parameters.
9. Measure weight daily.
10. Monitor arterial blood gases (ABGs), electrolyte levels, and serum osmolality.

V. Hyperosmolar Hyperglycemic Non-Ketotic Coma (HHNC)

A. **Description**
1. HHNC is characterized by a relative insulin deficiency (as opposed to DKA, in which an absolute insulin deficiency exists).
2. In HHNC, enough insulin is present to spare the body from accelerated fat metabolism; the result is hyperglycemia without ketonuria.
3. HHNC commonly occurs in patients with undiagnosed diabetes or in middle-aged patients with non–insulin-dependent diabetes mellitus.

 4. **HHNC is a life-threatening emergency presenting with severe hyperglycemia, hyperosmolar state and severe dehydration. There is minimal ketosis and often severe neurologic deficits.**

B. **Etiology**
1. Inadequate insulin secretion or action
2. Unintentional dietary indiscretions (eg, inadequate insulin intake)
3. Ingestion of certain medications (eg, thiazide diuretics, glucocorticoids, phenytoin, sympathomimetics)

C. **Pathophysiologic processes and clinical manifestations**
1. Not enough insulin is present to prevent hyperglycemia; however, enough is present to prevent ketonuria.
2. As a result of high serum glucose levels, glycosuria and poly-uria from osmotic diuresis occur.

3. Hyperglycemia increases osmolality of the ECF causing fluid to shift from ICF to ECF to balance high plasma osmolality. This causes intracellular dehydration, and results in severe neurologic symptoms such as coma.
4. Polyuria with electrolyte losses (from osmotic diuresis) results in dehydration of the ECF and ICF, causing neurologic changes.
5. The hyperglycemia of HHNC develops slower than DKA.

D. Overview of nursing interventions
   1. Monitor vital signs.
   2. Measure and record intake and output.
   3. **Monitor fluids and electrolyte status closely during treatment because intake is through intravenous route, the output is excessive, and electrolytes will shift as fluids are instilled.**
   4. Initiate fluid replacement with .9% NACL or .45% NACL to replenish the dehydrated ECF space. *There should be no potassium in the initial IV solutions because the potassium will shift from ICF to ECF as acidosis is corrected.*
   5. Administer insulin to correct hyperglycemia.

VI. Renal disease

A. Description
   1. Renal disease may be acute or chronic.
   2. Acute renal disease happens suddenly and is typically reversible.
   3. Chronic disease develops over a longer period of time and often is not reversible.

B. Etiology
   1. Renal diseases that can cause fluid and electrolyte imbalances are categorized according to three classifications.
   2. Pre-renal etiologies occur when there is an alteration in blood supply to the kidneys. Examples include renal ischemia from hypovolemia, aortic stenosis, blood clots, tumor obstruction to the renal vasculature, surgical clamping of the renal arteries of abdominal aorta above the level of these arteries (occurs with aneurysm repair).
   3. Intra-renal (also known as renal parenchymal) describes etiologies where the actual kidney tissue is damaged from a disease process such as diabetes, glomerulonephritis, hypertension, pyelonephritis.
   4. Post-renal failure (or obstructive uropathy) occurs when there is an obstruction to the flow of urine from the kidneys to the bladder. This obstruction causes urine to back up from the point of obstruction into the kidney pelvis and renal tissue. Examples include stones, tumors and congenital kinks.

C. Pathophysiologic processes and clinical manifestations
   1. **When the kidneys fail, no mechanism for maintaining fluid, electrolyte, and acid–base balance exists.**
   2. Depending on the mechanism of failure, damage occurs to the glomerulus or tubules, or both:
      a. Damage to the glomerulus hinders filtration capabilities, allowing excess fluids and electrolytes to pass.

        b.   Damage to the tubules causes them to become more or less permeable, resulting in altered elimination patterns.

   3. Damage to the glomerulus and filter also causes the buffer systems (protein, phosphate, bicarbonate) to fail, altering acid–base balance.

   4. Kidney damage also alters hormone secreting capabilities, affecting the levels of renin and erythropoietin:

        a.   Over-secretion of renin commonly occurs in renal failure, resulting in high blood pressure.

        b.   Inadequate erythropoietin secretion contributed to anemia before the hormone was available by parenteral preparation (Epogen).

   5. As acid waste products accumulate, they are unable to be buffered because the buffering mechanisms have failed.

   6. In low output states, fluid and electrolyte imbalances occur; these can include:

        a.   Hypervolemia
        b.   Hypernatremia
        c.   Hyperkalemia
        d.   Hypocalcemia
        e.   Hyperphosphatemia
        f.   Hypermagnesemia
        g.   Metabolic acidosis

   7. Hypervolemia can result in CHF or pulmonary edema.

   8. If the kidneys are not adequately perfused with blood, the nephrons will be damaged; as a result, the cause may be hard to distinguish from the effect if only output is evaluated.

D. **Overview of nursing interventions**

   1. Maintain accurate assessment of fluid balance by measuring and recording daily weights and intake and output and by closely monitoring vital signs, breath sounds, and hemodynamic parameters (if available).

   2. Be aware of signs of fluid overload (eg, dyspnea, rales, bounding pulse, edema, bulging neck veins).

   3. Monitor electrolyte levels because some electrolyte imbalances have deleterious effects.

   4. Monitor ABGs.

   5. Monitor electrocardiogram changes because disorders of potassium and calcium can cause cardiac dysrhythmia.

   6. Maintain dietary restrictions.

   7. Administer diuretics as ordered if the patient's kidneys are still able to eliminate urine.

   8. Administer bicarbonate as ordered if acidosis is severe; be aware that this may cause hypocalcemia because bicarbonate tends to bind calcium.

   9. Initiate dialysis if necessary.

VII. **GI fluid losses**

A. **Description: Excessive fluid losses (eg, intestinal secretions, gastric fluid, pancreatic juice) through the upper or lower GI tract**

B. **Etiology**

1. Viral or bacterial infection
2. Ulcers
3. Inflammatory diseases
4. Obstructions

5. **Surgical tubes**
6. Vomiting
7. Tube drainage

C.   Pathophysiologic processes and clinical manifestations

1. The types of fluid and electrolyte disorders that result from GI fluid losses depend on the amount and type of fluid lost.
2. Because fluids in the upper GI tract (eg, stomach, intestine, and pancreas) are rich in sodium, potassium, chloride, and hydrogen, upper GI losses tend to cause hypokalemia and metabolic alkalosis from loss of hydrogen.
3. Fluids in the lower GI tract are alkaline; as a result, acidosis commonly occurs when bases are lost due to diarrhea, fistulas, and ileostomies.

D.   Overview of nursing interventions

1. Measure and record intake and output carefully to track fluid losses.
2. Administer replacement solutions as ordered.
3. Assess fluid and electrolyte status.
4. Monitor ABGs.
5. Administer medications (eg, histamine 2-receptor antagonists, antacids, losec) as ordered.

VIII.   Respiratory dysfunction

A.   Description and etiology

1. The lungs play a critical role in maintaining the balance of CO_2 an acid.
2. Changes in the respiratory volume and rate (eg, hypoventilation or hyperventilation) alter the amount of CO_2 that is retained or excreted, resulting in respiratory acidosis or respiratory alkalosis.
3. *Hypoventilation* may result from:
   a. Central nervous system disorders (eg, stroke, head injury) in which the central stimulus to breathe is reduced by damage to the brain
   b. Respiratory disorders involving obstruction or fluid accumulation (eg, chronic obstructive pulmonary disorder, tumors, pulmonary edema, pneumonia)
   c. Cardiac disorders (eg, CHF)
4. *Hyperventilation* may result from:
   a. Tachypnea for any reason
   b. Inappropriate mechanical ventilation settings

B.   Pathophysiologic processes and clinical manifestations

1. Hypoventilation reduces oxygen delivery to the alveoli and CO_2 elimination, allowing retention of the acid CO_2.
2. As a result, respiratory acidosis occurs; ABG values reflect a low pH and a high CO_2.
3. Hyperventilation results in excess CO_2 elimination, leaving excess base (bi-

carbonate) in the blood and resulting in respiratory alkalosis; ABG values reflect high pH and low CO_2.

4. Patients who are mechanically ventilated may be hyperventilated or hypoventilated by inappropriate ventilator settings.

C. **Overview of nursing interventions**
   1. Monitor ABGs.
   2. Assess respiratory status.
   3. Administer oxygen as prescribed.
   4. Administer treatments to correct the cause of acidosis or alkalosis.

IX.   Decreased cardiac output

A. **Description: Inability of the heart to pump enough blood to perfuse the tissues and vital organs adequately; renal hypoperfusion results in FVE.**

B. **Etiology**
   1. CHF (may occur from volume expansion or pump failure)
   2. Cardiac depressant medication (eg, anesthetics)
   3. Cardiomyopathy
   4. Volume expansion
   5. Myocardial infarction

C. **Pathophysiologic processes and clinical manifestations**

   1. **As the heart's pumping ability fails, blood is unable to be ejected from the right ventricle to the lungs or from the left ventricle to the periphery.**
   2. The blood vessels then lose pressure (hypotension) because the pumping force is inadequate to propel the blood.
   3. Renal hypoperfusion, which can eventually cause prerenal azotemia, is sensed in the juxtaglomerular cells; in response, these cells secrete renin.
   4. The renin-angiotensin-aldosterone mechanism allows excess sodium to be reabsorbed in the kidney tubules.
   5. This sodium reabsorption also is accompanied by water reabsorption, exacerbating FVE.

   6. **Angiotensin causes massive vasoconstriction, forcing the heart to pump against the increased pressure, adding to afterload and exacerbating heart failure.**
   7. Total congestion of the heart's right or left side, or both sides, occurs.
   8. In right-sided heart failure, the ventricle is unable to eject blood into the aorta and through to the peripheral tissues; blood then backs up into the left atrium, pulmonary veins, and the pulmonary vasculature. Symptoms of right-sided heart failure include edema of the organs (eg, liver) and periphery (eg, feet, legs, and sacrum).
   9. In left-sided heart failure, the left ventricle is unable to eject blood from itself into the lungs; blood then backs up into the atrium, vena cava, and periphery. Symptoms of left-sided heart failure include manifestations of pulmonary edema:
      a. Rales at the bases
      b. Tachycardia

        c.   Hypoxia (due to pulmonary fluid accumulation)

        d.   Restlessness, diaphoresis, orthopnea, anuria, excessive pink secretions (these occur in the late stages)

10. If hypoperfusion is severe, metabolic acidosis results from excess lactic acid accumulation.

D. Overview of nursing interventions

1. Monitor fluid and electrolyte balance.

2. Monitor vital signs, EKG and hemodynamic parameters.

3. Provide a low-sodium diet.

4. Monitor pulmonary status closely, because life-threatening pulmonary edema can result.

5. Monitor serum electrolyte levels and ABGs.

6. Administer medications as prescribed to improve cardiac output.

7. Track daily weights because fluid increases are reflected in the daily weights (1 liter is approximately 2 pounds [1 kilogram]).

X. Burns

A. Description and etiology

1. Burns are traumatic injuries to the skin resulting from heat, electrical current, chemicals, friction, shearing forces, or excessive exposure to sunlight.

2. Fluid loss from burns is life-threatening.

3. Burns are classified according to the depth of destruction to the epidermis, dermis, or subcutaneous layers:

        a.   *First-degree* burn (partial thickness)

        b.   *Second-degree burn* (superficial or deep partial thickness)

        c.   *Third-degree burn* (full thickness)

B. Pathophysiologic processes and clinical manifestations

1. When the skin is burned, body fluids and electrolytes leak out.

2. The type and severity of the resultant fluid and electrolyte disorders depend on the extent of the burn; typically, severe burns pose the highest risk for significant disorders.

3. After a severe burn, edema accounts for some loss of plasma volume as fluid moves from the intravascular to the interstitial space and eventually to the intracellular space.

4. Water evaporation also occurs, further exacerbating fluid loss; this insensible loss cannot be measured and may be severe.

5. As plasma volume is lost, blood pressure drops, leading to poor perfusion of vital organs. Proteins and electrolytes also are lost. Blood loss may occur as well.

6. Decreased tissue perfusion produces lactic acid, causing metabolic acidosis.

7. Hypoventilation results in CO_2 retention, causing respiratory acidosis.

8. Because potassium is released whenever cells are destroyed, hyperkalemia can occur; it worsens if the burn is complicated by renal failure.

9. After 4 to 5 days, potassium may shift from the ECF to the ICF; extracellular FVE occurs as fluid shifts from the interstitial space into the intravascular space.

10. Hyponatremia occurs as large amounts of sodium are trapped in edema fluid. It also may result as fluids are remobilized.

D. **Overview of nursing interventions**

1. Administer IV fluid replacement therapy as ordered to restore depleted volume.
2. Assess cardiac, pulmonary, and fluid volume status.
3. Assess hemodynamic measurements to track the effectiveness of fluid volume replacement therapy.
4. Maintain patent airway if the upper airway is damaged from smoke inhalation.
5. Closely monitor the type and amount of fluids given because fluids and electrolytes will be lost through the skin and shift between compartments, affecting the well-being of the patient.

XI. Cirrhosis

A. **Description**

1. Cirrhosis is an irreversible chronic inflammatory disease characterized by massive degeneration and destruction of hepatocyte, resulting in a disorganized lobular pattern of regeneration.
2. Classifications of cirrhosis based on morphologic changes in regenerated nodules include micronodular cirrhosis, macro-nodular cirrhosis, and mixed cirrhosis.

B. **Etiology**

1. Alcoholism
2. Hepatotoxic medications
3. Blood transfusion reaction
4. Poor cardiac perfusion (right-sided CHF)
5. Biliary tract obstruction (strictures)
6. Complication of hepatitis

C. **Pathophysiologic processes and clinical manifestations**

1. Cirrhosis is a complicated disease, but it affects fluid and electrolyte balance in that liver damage prevents aldosterone and other hormones from metabolizing.
2. The presence of aldosterone leads to increased sodium reabsorption and subsequent potassium elimination (in some cases).
3. Water is reabsorbed along with sodium; the excess sodium and water tend to accumulate in the feet as pedal edema and in the abdomen as ascites.
4. Ascites results because of the poor metabolism of protein; when protein is present in the abdominal circulation as the blood exits the liver, it exerts its osmotic effect by drawing fluid into the peritoneal cavity.

D. **Overview of nursing interventions**

1. Administer spironolactone (Aldactone) as ordered to inhibit the sodium-retaining action of aldosterone; because sodium excretion is now possible, potassium will be retained, making hyperkalemia a possible complication.
2. Monitor the patient's amount of dietary protein intake, because patients with cirrhosis need more protein than others.
3. Measure abdominal girth daily to track the amount of fluid retained.

4. Monitor daily intake and output.
5. Measure and record daily weight.
6. Assess the patient for changes in cardiac output, decreased renal function, and electrolyte imbalances.

Bibliography

Bullock, B. (1996). *Pathophysiology: Adaptations and alterations in function* (4th ed.). Philadelphia: J. B. Lippincott.

Drummer, C., Gerzer, R., Heer, M., et al. (1992). Effects of an acute saline infusion on fluid and electrolyte metabolism in humans. *American Journal of Physiology,* May, 744–754.

Guyton, A. (1991). *Textbook of medical physiology* (8th ed.). Philadelphia: W. B. Saunders.

Kinney, M., Packa, D., & Dunbar, S. (1993). *AACN's clinical reference for critical-care nursing* (3rd ed.). St. Louis: C.V. Mosby.

Kokko, J., & Tannen, R. (1996). *Fluids and electrolytes* (3rd ed.). Philadelphia: W. B. Saunders.

Metheny, N. (1996). *Fluid and electrolyte balance: Nursing considerations* (3rd ed.). Philadelphia: J. B. Lippincott.

Miller, M. (1997). Fluid and electrolyte homeostasis in the elderly: physiologic changes of aging and clinical consequences. *Baillieres Clinical Endocrinology and Metabolism,* 11(2), 367–387.

Narrins, R. (Ed). (1994). *Maxwell & Kleemans clinical disorders of fluid and electrolyte metabolism* (5th ed.). New York: McGraw-Hill.

North American Nursing Diagnosis Association. Nursing Diagnosis: Definitions and Classifications. The Auth. 1996.

Plante, G. E., Chakir, M., Lehoux, S., & Lortie, M. (1995). Disorders of body fluid balance: A new look into the mechanisms of disease. *Canadian Journal of Cardiology,* 11(9), 788–802.

Porth, C. (1994). *Pathophysiology: Concepts of altered health states* (4th ed.). Philadelphia: J. B. Lippincott.

Rose, B. (1994). *Clinical physiology of acid-base and electrolyte disorders* (4th ed.). New York: McGraw-Hill.

Seaman, S. L. (1995). Renal physiology part II: Fluid and electrolyte regulation. *Neonatal network,* 14(5), 5–11.

Smith, K., & Brain, E. (1991). *Fluids and electrolytes: A conceptual approach* (2nd ed.). New York: Churchill Livingstone.

Szerlip, H., & Goldfarb, S. (1993). *Workshops in fluid and electrolyte disorders.* New York: Churchill Livingstone.

Toto, K. (1994). Endocrine physiology. *Critical Care Nursing Clinics of North America,* December, 647–657.

STUDY QUESTIONS

1. The mechanism by which hypoventilation results in acidosis involves:
   a. excretion of the acid CO_2
   b. retention of the acid CO_2
   c. retention of oxygen
   d. excretion of oxygen

2. The nurse would interpret a blood gas pH of 7.30 as indicating:
   a. acidosis
   b. alkalosis
   c. normal
   d. hypoxia

3. When assessing a patient with congestive heart failure (CHF), the nurse is aware that symptoms of left-sided heart failure include:
   a. sacral edema
   b. liver edema
   c. rales at the bases
   d. pedal edema

4. The nurse has provided patient teaching about dietary modifications for a patient with CHF. Which of the following menu selections indicates that the patient needs further education?
   a. corned beef sandwich
   b. fruit salad
   c. tuna salad sandwich
   d. bagel with butter

5. Nursing management of CHF includes:
   a. encouraging fluids
   b. keeping the head of the bed flat
   c. encouraging ambulation
   d. administering diuretics as ordered

6. Which of the following nursing diagnoses is consistent with diabetes insipidus?
   a. extracellular fluid volume deficit (FVD)
   b. intracellular fluid volume excess (FVE)
   c. extracellular FVE
   d. intracellular FVD

7. Metabolic acidosis occurs in diabetic ketoacidosis because:
   a. Aldosterone is an acid that is released.
   b. Lack of sugar causes acid release.
   c. Fat metabolism yields acid ketone bodies.
   d. Hyperventilation causes acid retention.

8. When estimating fluid loss, the nurse knows that fluid and electrolyte losses from severe burns occur through the skin and:
   a. blood vessels from bleeding
   b. fluid shifting and evaporation
   c. vomiting and diarrhea from shock
   d. all of the above

9. Which of the following acid–base imbalances is associated with burns?
   a. respiratory acidosis
   b. metabolic acidosis
   c. respiratory alkalosis
   d. metabolic alkalosis

10. Which electrolyte disorder occurs with SIADH?
    a. hyperkalemia
    b. hyponatremia
    c. hypercalcemia
    d. hypomagnesemia

11. Fluid and electrolyte imbalances occur with cirrhosis because of:
    a. poor metabolism of proteins and aldosterone
    b. renal disease that occurs early in the disease
    c. blood loss from esophageal varices
    d. the presence of ascites

ANSWER KEY

Question	Correct answer	Correct answer rationale	Incorrect answer rationales
1.	b	Hypoventilation reduces oxygen delivery to the alveoli and carbon dioxide elimination, allowing for retention of the acid CO_2 and acidosis.	a, c, and d. These choices do not reflect the mechanism resulting in acidosis.
2.	a	A pH lower then 7.35 indicates acidosis.	b. A pH greater than 7.45 indicates alkalosis. c. Normal pH is 7.35 to 7.45. d. Hypoxia is reflected in the oxygen mechanism, although the pH is effected the best choice is letter a.
3.	c	In left-sided CHF, fluid backs up into the lungs; symptoms include rales at the bases and hypoxia.	a, b, and d. These are symptoms of right-sided CHF.
4.	a	Corned beef contains high amounts of sodium, as do other smoked and preserved meats.	b, c, and d. These would be better menu selections.
5.	d	Treatment for a patient with CHF involves administering digoxin and diuretics, providing a low-sodium diet, keeping the head of the bed elevated, and encouraging bedrest.	a, b, and c. These are contraindicated in CHF.s
6.	a	Lack of antidiuretic hormone (ADH) allows excessive renal excretion of water, with liters being excreted each hour.	b. Intracellular FVE would be associated with a condition that produced sodium losses in excess of water. c. Extracellular FVE would be associated with a gain of water and salt. d. Intracellular FVD would be be associated with a gain of hypertonic solutions.
7.	c	Fat metabolism yields ketone bodies as an acid end-product, resulting in metabolic acidosis; fat metabolism occurs as the body uses fat for energy.	a. Aldosterone is a hormone, not an acid. b. This response is incorrect. d. Hyperventilation causes acid diminution, not retention.
8.	b	After a severe burn injury, edema accounts for some loss of plasma volume as fluid shifts occur. Water evaporation also occurs, increasing insensible fluid loss. Fluid shifting must always be accounted for when calculating fluid loss.	a and c. Fluid and electrolyte loss may occur via these routes, but not always.

Question	Correct answer	Correct answer rationale	Incorrect answer rationales
9.	b	Metabolic acidosis results as decreased tissue perfusion produces lactic acidosis.	a, c, and d. These acid–base disorders are not necessarily associated with burns.
10.	b	Hyponatremia occurs as excessive amounts of water is reabsorbed, diluting the ECF.	a, c, and d. These electrolyte disorders are not associated with SIADH.
11.	a	These two processes are primarily responsible for the fluid and electrolyte imbalances of cirrhosis.	b, c, and d. While Hepatomegaly, esophageal varices, and ascites occur they do not cause the fluid and electrolyte imbalances associated with ascites.

Comprehensive Test Questions

1. The nurse would interpret a serum chloride level of 96 mEq/L as:
   a. high
   b. low
   c. within normal range
   d. high normal

2. Which of the following conditions is associated with elevated serum chloride levels?
   a. cystitis
   b. diabetes
   c. eclampsia
   d. hypertension

3. In the extracellular fluid, chloride is a major:
   a. compound
   b. ion
   c. anion
   d. cation

4. Nursing interventions for the patient with hyperphosphatemia include encouraging intake of:
   a. amphogel
   b. Fleets phospho-soda
   c. milk
   e. vitamin D

5. Etiologies associated with hypocalcemia may include all of the following *except:*
   a. renal failure
   b. inadequate intake calcium
   c. metastatic bone lesions
   d. vitamin D deficiency

6. Which of the following findings would the nurse expect to assess in hypercalcemia?
   a. prolonged QRS complex
   b. tetany
   c. petechiae
   d. urinary calculi

7. Which of the following is not an appropriate nursing intervention for a patient with hypercalcemia?
   a. administering calcitonin
   b. administering calcium gluconate
   c. administering loop diuretics
   d. encouraging ambulation

8. A patient with which of the following disorders is at high risk to develop hypermagnesemia?
   a. insulin shock
   b. hyperadrenalism
   c. nausea and vomiting
   d. renal failure

9. Nursing interventions for a patient with hypermagnesemia include administering calcium gluconate to:
   a. increase calcium levels
   b. antagonize the cardiac effects of magnesium
   c. lower calcium levels
   d. lower magnesium levels

10. For a patient with hypomagnesemia, which of the following medications may become toxic?
    a. Lasix
    b. Digoxin
    c. calcium gluconate
    d. CAPD

11. Which of the following is the most important physical assessment parameter the nurse would consider when assessing fluid and electrolyte balance?
    a. skin turgor
    b. intake and output
    c. osmotic pressure
    d. cardiac rate and rhythm

12. Insensible fluid losses include:
    a. urine
    b. gastric drainage

c. bleeding
d. perspiration

13. Which of the following intravenous solutions would be appropriate for a patient with severe hyponatremia secondary to syndrome of inappropriate antidiuretic hormone (SIADH)?
   a. hypotonic solution
   b. hypertonic solution
   c. isotonic solution
   d. normotonic solution

14. Aldosterone secretion in response to fluid loss will result in which one of the following electrolyte imbalances?
   a. hypokalemia
   b. hyperkalemia
   c. hyponatremia
   d. hypernatremia

15. When assessing a patient for signs of fluid overload, the nurse would expect to observe:
   a. bounding pulse
   b. flat neck veins
   c. poor skin turgor
   d. vesicular

16. The physician has ordered IV replacement of potassium for a patient with severe hypokalemia. The nurse would administer this:
   a. by rapid bolus
   b. diluted in 100 cc over 1 hour
   c. diluted in 10 cc over 10 minutes
   d. IV push

17. Which of the following findings would the nurse expect to assess in a patient with hypokalemia?
   a. hypertension
   b. pH below 7.35
   c. hypoglycemia
   d. hyporeflexia

18. Oral potassium supplements should be administered:
   a. undiluted
   b. diluted
   c. on an empty stomach
   d. at bedtime

19. Normal venous blood pH ranges from:

a. 6.8 to 7.2
b. 7.31 to 7.41
c. 7.35 to 7.45
d. 7.0 to 8.0

20. Respiratory regulation of acids and bases involves:
   a. hydrogen
   b. hydroxide
   c. oxygen
   d. carbon dioxide

21. To determine if a patient's respiratory system is functioning, the nurse would assess which of the following parameters:
   a. respiratory rate
   b. pulse
   c. arterial blood gas
   d. pulse oximetry

22. Which of the following conditions is an equal decrease of extracellular fluid (ECF) solute and water volume?
   a. hypotonic FVD
   b. isotonic FVD
   c. hypertonic FVD
   d. isotonic FVE

23. When monitoring the daily weight of a patient with fluid volume deficit (FVD), the nurse is aware that fluid loss may be considered when weight loss begins to exceed:
   a. 0.25 lb
   b. 0.50 lb
   c. 1 lb
   d. 1 kg

24. Dietary recommendations for a patient with a hypotonic fluid excess should include:
   a. decreased sodium intake
   b. increased sodium intake
   c. increased fluid intake
   d. intake of potassium-rich foods

25. Osmotic pressure is created through the process of:
   a. osmosis
   b. diffusion
   c. filtration
   d. capillary dynamics

26. A rise in arterial pressure causes the baroreceptors and stretch receptors to signal an inhibition of the sympathetic nervous system, resulting in:
    a. decreased sodium reabsorption
    b. increased sodium reabsorption
    c. decreased urine output
    d. increased urine output

27. Normal serum sodium concentration ranges from:
    a. 120 to 125 mEq/L
    b. 125 to 130 mEq/L
    c. 136 to 145 mEq/L
    d. 140 to 148 mEq/L

28. When assessing a patient for electrolyte balance, the nurse is aware that etiologies for hyponatremia include:
    a. water gain
    b. diuretic therapy
    c. diaphoresis
    d. all of the following

29. Nursing interventions for a patient with hyponatremia include:
    a. administering hypotonic IV fluids
    b. encouraging water intake
    c. restricting fluid intake
    d. restricting sodium intake

30. The nurse would analyze an arterial pH of 7.46 as indicating:
    a. acidosis
    b. alkalosis
    c. homeostasis
    d. neutrality

31. The net diffusion of water from one solution through a semipermeable membrane to another solution containing a lower concentration of water is termed:
    a. filtration
    b. diffusion
    c. osmosis
    d. brownian motion

32. When assessing a patient's total body water percentage, the nurse is aware that all of the following factors influence this *except:*
    a. age
    b. fat tissue
    c. muscle mass
    d. gender

33. Which of the following symptoms would the nurse expect to assess in a patient with fluid volume deficit (FVD)?
    a. rales
    b. bounding pulse
    c. tachycardia
    d. bulging neck veins

34. Nursing management of a patient receiving hypertonic fluids includes monitoring for all of the following potential complications *except:*
    a. water intoxication
    b. fluid volume excess (FVE)
    c. cellular dehydration
    d. cell shrinkage

35. A patient is scheduled to receive an isotonic solution; which one of the following solutions could cause harm?
    a. D10% W
    b. 0.45% saline
    c. 0.9% saline
    d. 3% normal salineW

36. Which of the following arterial blood gas (ABG) values indicates uncompensated metabolic alkalosis?
    a. pH 7.48, $PaCO_2$ 42, HCO_3 30
    b. pH 7.48, $PaCO_2$ 46, HCO_3 30
    c. pH 7.48, $PaCO_2$ 34, HCO_3 20
    d. pH 7.48, $PaCO_2$ 34, HCO_3 26

37. The body's compensation of metabolic alkalosis involves:
    a. increasing the respiratory rate
    b. decreasing the respiratory rate
    c. increasing urine output
    d. decreasing urine output

38. When assessing a patient for metabolic alkalosis, the nurse would expect to find:
    a. low serum potassium
    b. changes in urine output
    c. hypotension
    d. increased CVP

39. Which of the following blood products should be infused rapidly?
    a. packed red blood cells (PRBC)

b. fresh frozen plasma (FFP)
c. platelets
d. dextran

40. Which of the following statements provides the rationale for using a hypotonic solution for a patient with FVD?
   a. A hypotonic solution provides free water to help the kidneys eliminate the solute.
   b. A hypotonic solution supplies an excess of sodium and chloride ions.
   c. Excessive volumes are recommended in the early postoperative period.
   d. A hypotonic solution is used to treat hyponatremia.

41. When monitoring a patient who is receiving a blood transfusion, the nurse would analyze an elevated body temperature as indicating:
   a. a normal physiologic process
   b. evidence of sepsis
   c. a possible transfusion reaction
   d. an expected response to the transfusion

42. The process of endocrine regulation of electrolytes involves:
   a. sodium reabsorption and chloride excretion
   b. chloride reabsorption and sodium excretion
   c. potassium reabsorption and sodium excretion
   d. sodium reabsorption and potassium excretion

43. The chief anion in the intracellular fluid (ICF) is:
   a. phosphorus
   b. potassium
   c. sodium
   d. chloride

44. The major cation in the ICF is:
   a. potassium
   b. sodium
   c. phosphorus
   d. magnesium

45. Hypophosphatemia may result from which of the following diseases?
   a. liver cirrhosis
   b. renal failure
   c. Paget's disease
   d. alcoholism

46. A patient with which of the following disorders is at high risk for developing hyperphosphatemia?
   a. hyperkalemia
   b. hyponatremia
   c. hypocalcemia
   d. hyperglycemia

47. Normal calcium levels must be analyzed in relation to:
   a. sodium
   b. glucose
   c. protein
   d. fats

48. Calcium is absorbed in the GI tract under the influence of:
   a. vitamin D
   b. glucose
   c. HCl
   d. vitamin C

49. Which of the following nursing diagnoses is most appropriate for a patient with hypocalcemia?
   a. constipation, bowel
   b. high risk for injury: bleeding
   c. airway clearance, ineffective
   d. high risk for injury: confusion

50. When serum calcium levels rise, which of the following hormones is secreted?
   a. aldosterone
   b. renin
   c. parathyroid hormone
   d. calcitonin

51. The presence of which of the following electrolytes contributes to acidosis?
   a. sodium
   b. potassium
   c. hydrogen
   d. chloride

52. The lungs participate in acid–base balance by:

a. reabsorbing bicarbonate
b. splitting carbonic acid in two
c. using CO_2 to regulate hydrogen ions
d. sending hydrogen ions to the renal tubules

53. The respiratory system regulates acid–base balance by:
    a. increasing mucus production
    b. changing the rate and depth of respirations
    c. forming bicarbonate
    d. reabsorbing bicarbonate

54. Which of the following is a gas component of the ABG measurement?
    a. carbon dioxide
    b. bicarbonate
    c. hydrogen
    d. pH

55. Chloride helps maintain acid–base balance by performing which of the following roles?
    a. participating in the chloride shift
    b. following sodium to maintain serum osmolarity
    c. maintaining the balance of cations in the ICF and ECF
    d. separating carbonic acid

56. Which of the following hormones helps regulate chloride reabsorption?
    a. antidiuretic hormone (ADH)
    b. renin
    c. estrogen
    d. aldosterone

57. Chloride is absorbed in the:
    a. stomach
    b. bowel
    c. liver
    d. kidney

58. When chloride concentration drops below 95 mEq/L, reabsorption of which of the following electrolytes increases proportionally?
    a. hydrogen
    b. potassium
    c. sodium
    d. bicarbonate

59. A patient is admitted with 1,000 ml of diarrhea per day for the last 3 days. An IV of 0.45% NaCl mixed with 5% dextrose is infusing. Which of the following nursing interventions is the most appropriate?
    a. Get an infusion controller from central supply.
    b. Mix all antibiotics in 0.45% NaCl with 5% dextrose.
    c. Check the patient's potassium level and contact the doctor for IV additive orders.
    d. Assess the patient for signs of hyperkalemia.

60. Mrs. Jones is receiving digoxin and Lasix daily. Today, Mrs. Jones complains of nausea, and her apical pulse is 130 and irregular. Which of the following nursing interventions is the most appropriate?
    a. Hold the digoxin and check the patient's potassium level.
    b. Remove the orange juice from the patient's tray.
    c. Identify the patient as high risk for hyperkalemia.
    d. Assess the patient for other signs of hypernatremia.

61. The type of fluid used to manipulate fluid shifts among compartments states is:
    a. whole blood
    b. TPN
    c. albumin
    d. Ensure

62. Marathon runners are at high risk for fluid volume deficit. Which one of the following is a related factor?
    a. decreased diuresis
    b. disease-related processes
    c. decreased breathing and perspiration
    d. increased breathing and perspiration

63. A patient has a nursing diagnosis of fluid volume deficit. Which one of the following medications could potentially exacerbate the problem?

a. Synthroid
b. Digoxin
c. Lasix
d. insulin

64. In renal regulation of water balance, the functions of angiotensin II include:
    a. blood clotting within the nephron
    b. increasing progesterone secretion into the renal tubules
    c. catalyzing calcium-rich nutrients
    d. selectively constricting portions of the arteriole in the nephron

65. The majority of gastrointestinal reabsorption of water occurs in:
    a. the small intestines
    b. the esophagus
    c. the colon
    d. the stomach

66. Etiologies associated with hypomagnesemia include:
    a. decreased vitamin D intake
    b. constipation
    c. malabsorption syndrome
    d. renal failure

67. Magnesium performs all of the following functions *except:*
    a. contributing to vasoconstriction
    b. assisting in cardiac muscle contraction
    c. facilitating sodium transport
    d. assisting in protein metabolism

68. Magnesium reabsorption is controlled by:
    a. Loop of Henle
    b. glomerulus
    c. pituitary
    d. parathyroid hormone

69. Symptoms of hypermagnesemia may include:
    a. hypertension
    b. tachycardia
    c. hyperactive deep-tendon reflexes
    d. cardiac arrhythmias

70. When teaching a patient about foods high in magnesium, the nurse would include:

a. green vegetables
b. butter
c. cheese
d. tomatoes

71. Which of the following nursing diagnoses might apply to a patient with isotonic FVD?
    a. altered urinary elimination
    b. decreased cardiac output
    c. increased cardiac output
    d. ineffective airway clearance

72. Which of the following findings would the nurse expect to assess in a patient with hypotonic FVE?
    a. poor skin turgor and increased thirst
    b. weight gain and thirst
    c. interstitial edema and hypertension
    d. hypotension and pitting edema

73. Which of the following nursing diagnoses might apply to a patient with hypertonic FVE?
    a. ineffective airway clearance
    b. potential for decreased cardiac output
    c. ineffective breathing pattern
    d. potential for increased cardiac output

74. Isotonic FVD can result from:
    a. GI fluid loss through diarrhea
    b. insensible water loss during prolonged fever
    c. inadequate ingestion of fluids and electrolytes
    d. impaired thirst regulation

75. The danger of fluid sequestered in the third space is that the fluid:
    a. is hypertonic and can cause hypervolemia
    b. is hypotonic and can cause water intoxication
    c. is not available for circulation
    d. contains large amounts of acids

76. Which of the following clinical conditions exacerbates electrolyte excretion?
    a. nasogastric feedings

b. use of surgical drains
c. immobility from fractures
d. chronic water drinking

77. Which of the following electrolytes are lost as a result of vomiting?
   a. bicarbonate and calcium
   b. sodium and hydrogen
   c. sodium and potassium
   d. hydrogen and potassium

78. Bicarbonate is lost during which of the following clinical conditions?
   a. diarrhea
   b. diuresis
   c. diaphoresis
   d. vomiting

79. Disease of which of the following structures is most likely to affect electrolyte reabsorption?
   a. glomerulus
   b. renal tubules
   c. bladder
   d. renal pelvis

80. The balance of anions to cations as it occurs across cell membranes is known as:
   a. osmotic activity
   b. electrical neutrality
   c. electrical stability
   d. sodium–potassium pump

81. Body fluids perform which of the following functions?
   a. transport nutrients
   b. transport electrical charges
   c. cushion the organs
   d. facilitate fat metabolism

82. The interstitial space holds approximately how many liters?
   a. 3 L
   b. 6 L
   c. 9 L
   d. 12 L

83. The intracellular compartment holds water and:
   a. proteins
   b. glucose
   c. sodium
   d. uric acid

84. The majority of the body's water is contained in which of the following fluid compartments?
   a. intracellular
   b. interstitial
   c. intravascular
   d. extracellular

85. The extracellular fluid space holds water, electrolytes, proteins and:
   a. red blood cells
   b. potassium
   c. lipids
   d. nucleic acids

86. A diet containing the minimum daily sodium requirement for an adult would be:
   a. a no-salt-added diet
   b. a diet including 2 gm sodium
   c. a diet including 4 gm sodium
   d. a 1500 calorie weight-loss diet

87. Sodium balance is important for which of the following functions?
   a. transmitting impulses in nerve and muscle fibers via the calcium–potassium pump
   b. exchanging for magnesium and attracting chloride
   c. combining with hydrogen and chloride for acid-base balance
   d. exchanging for potassium and attracting chloride

88. Sodium levels are affected by the secretion of which of the following hormones?
   a. progesterone and aldosterone
   b. ADH and ACTH
   c. antidiuretic hormone and FSH
   d. ECF and aldosterone

89. An 85-year-old patient with a feeding tube has been experiencing severe watery stool. The patient is lethargic and has poor skin turgor, a pulse of 120, and hyperactive reflexes. Nursing interventions would include:
   a. measuring and recording intake and output and daily weights
   b. administering salt tablets and monitoring hypertonic parenteral solutions

c. administering sedatives

d. applying wrist restraints to avoid displacement of the feeding tube

90. A patient with a diagnosis of bipolar disorder has been drinking copious amounts of water and voiding frequently. The patient is experiencing muscle cramps, twitching, and is reporting dizziness. The nurse checks lab work for:

a. complete blood count results, particularly the platelets

b. electrolytes, particularly the serum sodium

c. urine analysis, particularly for the presence of white blood cells

d. EEG results

91. When recording a patient's intake, the nurse would include:

a. 120 cc of juice, 1 cup of mashed potatoes, and 700 cc IV solution

b. 500 cc of tube feeding, 60 cc of lactulose by mouth, and 750 cc IV solution

c. 1 hamburger, 1/2 cup of carrots, and 1 cup of ice cream

d. 750 cc IV solution, 1 cup of ice cream, and 1 cup of tapioca pudding

92. When assessing a patient's intake and output, the nurse would note the following abnormal findings:

a. decreased urine output and the presence of edema

b. weight gain and dyspnea

c. rapid pulse and decreased urine output

d. distended jugular vein and tachycardia

93. A cancer patient comes to the emergency department complaining of a high fever. The patient states, "I've been sweating a lot, and I'm really thirsty." The nurse explains that:

a. "Due to the fever, you have lost fluid by sweating and your body is trying to compensate by getting you to take in more fluids."

b. "Your sweaty and thirsty because

you have been really hot. It will pass when the fever is over."

c. "Fever doesn't usually cause sweating and thirst. Has there been something else going on?"

d. "This is just a side effect of your chemotherapy. When you finish your treatment, it will go away."

94. Which of the following medical problems would place a patient at risk for metabolic acidosis?

a. retention of bicarbonate

b. lactic acid deficit

c. aspirin overdose

d. constipation

95. Which of the following series of assessment findings indicate respiratory alkalosis?

a. dizziness, an excited state, and flaccid muscles

b. high serum potassium, flaccid muscles, and paresthesia

c. low serum potassium, confusion, and paresthesia

d. high serum chloride, low serum potassium, and dizziness

96. The nurse is caring for a patient with IV orders for lactated Ringer's solution to infuse at 100 cc's per hour. When doing the first assessment, the nurse would:

a. Check that the ordered solution is hanging and the flow rate is within 2 hours.

b. Check the the ordered solution is hanging and the flow rate is accurate.

c. Discontinue the infusion after 100 cc's have infused.

d. Check the IV site only.

97. The nurse assesses a patient's IV site and finds that it is red, hot, and tender to touch. The most appropriate first action is:

a. Stop the infusion and remove the IV.

b. Apply a warm soak to the site and reevaluate.

c. Stop the infusion and restart the IV in the same area.

d. Call the physician to evaluate.

98. In a severe burn, which elecrolyte shifts from the ECF to the ICF?

a. sodium

b. potassium

c. magnesium

d. chloride

99. Sodium and potassium levels are altered in cirrhosis because of the presence of:

a. antidiuretic hormone (ADH)

b. nitrogen

c. aldosterone

d. ammonia

100. In SIADH, water intake should be:

a. encouraged

b. restricted

c. no change in water intake

d. given intravenously

Answer Sheet for Comprehensive Test Questions

With a pencil, blacken the circle under the option you have chosen for your correct answer.

	A	B	C	D		A	B	C	D		A	B	C	D
1.	○	○	○	○	21.	○	○	○	○	41.	○	○	○	○
2.	○	○	○	○	22.	○	○	○	○	42.	○	○	○	○
3.	○	○	○	○	23.	○	○	○	○	43.	○	○	○	○
4.	○	○	○	○	24.	○	○	○	○	44.	○	○	○	○
5.	○	○	○	○	25.	○	○	○	○	45.	○	○	○	○
6.	○	○	○	○	26.	○	○	○	○	46.	○	○	○	○
7.	○	○	○	○	27.	○	○	○	○	47.	○	○	○	○
8.	○	○	○	○	28.	○	○	○	○	48.	○	○	○	○
9.	○	○	○	○	29.	○	○	○	○	49.	○	○	○	○
10.	○	○	○	○	30.	○	○	○	○	50.	○	○	○	○
11.	○	○	○	○	31.	○	○	○	○	51.	○	○	○	○
12.	○	○	○	○	32.	○	○	○	○	52.	○	○	○	○
13.	○	○	○	○	33.	○	○	○	○	53.	○	○	○	○
14.	○	○	○	○	34.	○	○	○	○	54.	○	○	○	○
15.	○	○	○	○	35.	○	○	○	○	55.	○	○	○	○
16.	○	○	○	○	36.	○	○	○	○	56.	○	○	○	○
17.	○	○	○	○	37.	○	○	○	○	57.	○	○	○	○
18.	○	○	○	○	38.	○	○	○	○	58.	○	○	○	○
19.	○	○	○	○	39.	○	○	○	○	59.	○	○	○	○
20.	○	○	○	○	40.	○	○	○	○	60.	○	○	○	○

	A	B	C	D		A	B	C	D		A	B	C	D
61.	○	○	○	○	81.	○	○	○	○	101.	○	○	○	○
62.	○	○	○	○	82.	○	○	○	○	102.	○	○	○	○
63.	○	○	○	○	83.	○	○	○	○	103.	○	○	○	○
64.	○	○	○	○	84.	○	○	○	○	104.	○	○	○	○
65.	○	○	○	○	85.	○	○	○	○	105.	○	○	○	○
66.	○	○	○	○	86.	○	○	○	○	106.	○	○	○	○
67.	○	○	○	○	87.	○	○	○	○	107.	○	○	○	○
68.	○	○	○	○	88.	○	○	○	○	108.	○	○	○	○
69.	○	○	○	○	89.	○	○	○	○	109.	○	○	○	○
70.	○	○	○	○	90.	○	○	○	○	110.	○	○	○	○
71.	○	○	○	○	91.	○	○	○	○	111.	○	○	○	○
72.	○	○	○	○	92.	○	○	○	○	112.	○	○	○	○
73.	○	○	○	○	93.	○	○	○	○	113.	○	○	○	○
74.	○	○	○	○	94.	○	○	○	○	114.	○	○	○	○
75.	○	○	○	○	95.	○	○	○	○	115.	○	○	○	○
76.	○	○	○	○	96.	○	○	○	○	116.	○	○	○	○
77.	○	○	○	○	97.	○	○	○	○	117.	○	○	○	○
78.	○	○	○	○	98.	○	○	○	○	118.	○	○	○	○
79.	○	○	○	○	99.	○	○	○	○	119.	○	○	○	○
80.	○	○	○	○	100.	○	○	○	○	120.	○	○	○	○

Comprehensive Test
Answer Key

Question	Correct answer	Correct answer rationale	Incorrect answer rationales
1.	c	Normal serum concentrations of chloride range from 95 to 208 mEq/L.	a. High chloride levels are above 108 mEq/L. b. Low chloride levels are below 95 mEq/L. d. A chloride level of 96 is on the low border of normal.
2.	c	Eclampsia is associated with decreased levels of serum chloride.	a, b, and d. Cystitis, diabetes, and hypertension are not associated with decreased levels of serum chloride.
3.	c	Chloride is a major anion found in extracellular fluid.	a. A compound occurs when two ions are bound together. b. Chloride is an ion, but this is too general an answer. d. HCO_3 is a cation.
4.	a	Administration of phosphate binders (amphogel and basagel) will reduce the serum phosphate levels.	b, c, and d. Fleets phospho-soda, milk, and vitamin D will increase serum phosphate levels.
5.	c	Metastatic bone lesions are associated with hypercalcemia due to accelerated bone metabolism and release of calcium into the serum.	a, b, and d. Renal failure, inadequate calcium intake, and vitamin D deficiency may cause hypocalcemia.
6.	d	Urinary calculi may occur with hypercalcemia.	a. Shortened, not prolonged QRS complex would be seen in hypercalcemia. b and c. Tetany and petechiae are signs of hypocalcemia.
7.	b	Calcium gluconate is used for replacement in deficiency states.	a and c. Calcitonin and loop diuretics are administered to lower serum calcium. d. Ambulation is recommended to prevent the movement of calcium from the bone.
8.	d	Renal failure can reduce magnesium excretion, leading to hypermagnesemia.	a. Diabetic ketoacidosis, not insulin shock is a cause of hypermagnesemia. b. Hypoadrenalism, not hyperadrenalism is a cause of hypermagnesemia. c. Nausea and vomiting lead to hypomagnesemia.

Question	Correct answer	Correct answer rationale	Incorrect answer rationales
9.	b	In a patient with hypermagnesemia, administration of calcium gluconate will antagonize the cardiac effects of magnesium.	a. Although calcium gluconate will raise serum calcium levels, that is not the purpose for its administration. c and d. Calcium gluconate does not lower calcium or magnesium levels.
10.	b	In hypomagnesemia, a patient on digoxin is likely to develop digitalis toxicity.	a and c. Neither of these medications has toxicity as a side effect. d. CAPD is not a medication.
11.	d	Cardiac rate and rhythm are the most important physical assessment parameter to measure.	a and b. Skin turgor, intake and output are physical assessment parameters the nurse would consider when assessing fluid and electrolyte balance, but choice d is the most important. c. Osmotic pressure is the phenomenon which causes fluids to move in both directions simultaneously; it is not a parameter that is assessed.
12.	d	Perspiration and the fluid lost via the lungs are termed insensible losses; normally, insensible losses equal about 1000 cc/day.	a, b, and c. These types of fluid losses are measurable and therefore are *not* insensible.
13.	b	When hyponatremia is severe, hypertonic solutions may be used but should be infused with caution due to the potential for development of CHF.	a and c. In SIADH, hypotonic and isotonic solutions are not indicated because urine output is minimal, so water is retained. This water retention dilutes serum sodium levels, making the patient hyponatremic and necessitating administration of hypertonic solutions to balance sodium and water. d. Normotonic solutions do not exist.
14.	a	Aldosterone is secreted in response to fluid loss. Aldosterone causes sodium reabsorption and potassium elimination, further exacerbating hypokalemia.	b, c, and d. Hyperkalemia, hyponatremia, and hypernatremia do not result from aldosterone secretion.
15.	a	Bounding pulse is a sign of fluid overload as more volume in the vessels causes a stronger sensation against the blood vessel walls.	b and d. Flat neck veins, and vesicular breath sounds are normal findings. c. Poor skin turgor is consistent with dehydration.
16.	b	Potassium must be well diluted and given slowly because rapid administration will cause cardiac arrest.	a, c, and d. Potassium must *never* be administered rapidly as a bolus because cardiac arrest will result.

Question	Correct answer	Correct answer rationale	Incorrect answer rationales
17.	d	Hyporeflexia is a symptom of hypo-kalemia.	a, b, and c. Hypotension, pH above 7.45, and hyperglycemia are symptoms of hypokalemia.
18.	b	Oral potassium supplements are known to irritate gastrointestinal (GI) mucosa and should be diluted.	a, c, and d. When taken undiluted, on an empty stomach, or at bedtime (when the stomach is empty), oral potassium supplements will cause GI irritation.
19.	b	Normal venous blood pH ranges from 7.31 to 7.41.	a and d. These are not normal pH values. c. Normal arterial blood pH ranges from 7.35 to 7.45.
20.	d	Respiratory regulation of acid–base balance involves the elimination or retention of carbon dioxide.	a, b, and c. Oxygen, hydrogen, and hydroxide are not involved in the respiratory regulation of acid–base balance.
21.	c	Arterial blood gases will indicate CO_2 and O_2 levels. This is an indication that the respiratory system is functioning.	a. Respiratory rate can reveal data about other systems, such as the brain, making letter c a better choice. b. Pulse rate is not measure of respiratory status. d. Pulse oximetry yields oxygen saturation levels, which is not a measure of acid–base balance.
22.	b	Isotonic FVD involves an equal decrease in solute concentration and water volume.	a, c, and d. These conditions produce different changes in the solute concentration and water volume.
23.	b	Weight loss of more than 0.50 lb. is considered to be fluid loss.	a. Weight loss of 0.25 lb is not significant enough to be considered fluid loss. c and d. Although 1 lb and 1 kg could be considered fluid loss, the nurse would begin to identify fluid loss with a weight loss of 0.50 lb.
24.	b	Hypotonic fluid volume excess (FVE) involves an increase in water volume without an increase in sodium concentration. Increased sodium intake is part of the management of this condition.	a. Decreased sodium intake will exacerbate the condition, since hypotonic FVE is associated with low sodium. c. Fluids are restricted, not increased. d. Intake of potassium-rich foods is not related to hypotonic FVE.
25.	b	In diffusion, the solute moves from an area of higher concentration to one of lower concentration, creating osmotic pressure.	a. Osmotic pressure is related to the process of osmosis. c. Filtration is created by hydrostatic pressure. d. Capillary dynamics are related to fluid exchange at the intravascular and interstitial levels.

Question	Correct answer	Correct answer rationale	Incorrect answer rationales
26.	d	Arterial baroreceptors and stretch receptors help maintain fluid balance by increasing urine output in response to a rise in arterial pressure.	a and b. Decreased or increased sodium reabsorption occurs in response to the secretion of the atrial natriuretic factor. c. Increased, not decreased urine output occurs.
27.	c	Normal serum sodium level ranges from 136 to 145 mEq/L.	a, b, and d. These are not normal sodium levels.
28.	d	Water gain, diuretic therapy, and diaphoresis are etiologies of hyponatremia.	
29.	c	Hyponatremia involves a decreased concentration of sodium in relation to fluid volume, so restricting fluid intake is indicated.	a. Hypotonic fluids will exacerbate hyponatremia. b. Fluids are restricted, not encouraged. d. Sodium intake is restricted, not encouraged.
30.	b	Alkalosis is indicated by a pH above 7.45.	a. Acidosis is indicated by a pH below 7.35. c. Homeostasis is present when a normal pH is present. d. Neutrality is the pH range from 7.35 to 7.45.
31.	c	Osmosis is defined as the diffusion of water through a semipermeable membrane to a solution with a lower concentration of water.	a. Filtration is the process in which fluids are pushed through biologic membranes by unequal processes. b and d. Diffusion (brownian motion) is the random kinetic motion causing atoms and molecules to spread out evenly.
32.	d	A patient's gender does not influence the percentage of total body water.	a, b, and c. A patient's age and amount of fat tissue and lean muscle do influence the percentage of total body water.
33.	c	Tachycardia, poor tissue turgor, and hypotension are symptoms of FVD.	a, b, and d. Rales, bounding pulse, and bulging neck veins are symptoms of FVE.
34.	a	Water intoxication is a potential complication associated with hypotonic fluid administration.	b, c, and d. FVE, cellular dehydration, and cell shrinkage are potential complications of hypertonic fluid administration.
35.	c	A solution of 0.9% saline is isotonic.	a, b, and d. Solutions of 0.33% and 0.45% saline and D_5W are hypotonic (eg, osmolar concentration is lower than plasma).
36.	a	Uncompensated metabolic alkalosis is indicated by ABG values of pH 7.48, $PaCO_2$ 42, and HCO_3 30.	b. These ABG values indicate metabolic alkalosis, partially compensated.

Question	Correct answer	Correct answer rationale	Incorrect answer rationales
			c. These ABG values indicate respiratory alkalosis, partially compensated. d. These ABG values indicate respiratory alkalosis, uncompensated.
37.	b	The body attempts to compensate for metabolic alkalosis by decreasing the respiratory rate and conserving carbon dioxide (an acid).	a. This response is incorrect. c and d. Urine volume does not influence acid–base balance.
38.	a	Decreased serum potassium is a common symptom of metabolic alkalosis	A change in urinary status, hypotension, and increased CVP are not symptoms of metabolic alkalosis.
39.	c	Platelets and cryoprecipitate can be infused quickly.	a and b. PRBC and FFP should be administered over 1 1/2 to 4 hours. d. Dextran is not a blood product.
40.	a	Hypotonic solutions provide free water, which helps the kidneys eliminate solute.	b. Hypotonic solutions are poor sources of sodium and chloride ions. c. Excessive volumes are not recommended in early postoperative periods since stress can increase ADH secretion. d. Hypertonic solutions are used to treat hyponatremia.
41.	c	An increase in body temperature indicates a possible transfusion reaction and requires immediate discontinuation of the infusion.	b. There is inadequate evidence for sepsis to be considered. a and d. An elevated body temperature is neither a normal nor an expected finding.
42.	d	ACTH stimulates release of aldosterone, which in turn acts on the tubules to reabsorb sodium. When this occurs, the cation potassium is excreted.	a and b. Chloride is not involved in this process. c. Potassium reabsorption is not influenced by the endocrine system.
43.	a	Phosphorus is the chief anion found in the ICF.	c and b. Potassium and sodium are cations. d. Chloride is the chief anion found in the ECF.
44.	a	Potassium is the major ICF cation.	b. Sodium is the major ECF cation c. Phosphorus is the major ICF anion. d. Magnesium is the second-most abundant cation in the ICF.
45.	d	Hypophosphatemia may occur secondary to alcoholism.	a and c. Liver cirrhosis and Paget's disease generally have no effect on phosphorous levels. b. Renal failure is usually associated with hyperphosphatemia.

Question	Correct answer	Correct answer rationale	Incorrect answer rationales
46.	c	Because calcium and phosphorous ratios are inversely proportional, when phosphorous levels are high, calcium levels are low.	a, b, and d. These conditions have no influence on phosphorous levels.
47.	c	Some calcium is bound to protein, so abnormal calcium levels are analyzed in relation to proteins.	a, b, and d. Sodium, glucose, and fats are not related to calcium levels.
48.	a	Calcium is absorbed in the GI tract under the influence of vitamin D in its biologically active form.	b, c, and d. Calcium reabsorption is not related to these elements in any way.
49.	b	A patient with hypocalcemia may bleed, since calcium is required for normal blood clotting.	a and d. These nursing diagnoses are appropriate for a patient with hypercalcemia. c. Ineffective airway clearing is not associated with fluctuating calcium levels.
50.	d	When calcium levels rise, calcitonin is secreted from the thyroid; this hormone moves calcium from plasma into bone.	a and b. These hormones are not secreted in response to calcium levels. c. Parathyroid hormone is secreted in response to lowered calcium levels; this hormone moves calcium from bone into plasma.
51.	c	The presence of hydrogen ions determines a solution's acidity.	a, b, and d. These ions do not influence a solution's acidity or alkalinity.
52.	c	The lungs use carbon dioxide to regulate hydrogen ion concentration.	a, b, and d. These are not actions that the lungs perform.
53.	b	Through changes in the rate and depth of respirations, acid–base balance is achieved via CO_2 elimination and retention.	a. Mucus production is not part of the pulmonary regulatory system. c and d. These responses refer to ways in which the kidneys balance acids and bases.
54.	a	The gases measured by ABGs are oxygen and carbon dioxide.	b, c, and d. Bicarbonate and hydrogen are ions; their ratio is measured in the pH.
55.	a	To maintain acid–base balance, chloride shifts into and out of red blood cells in exchange for bicarbonate.	b and c. Although these are roles of chloride, they do not help balance acids and bases. d. Chloride does not act to separate carbonic acid.
56.	d	Chloride reabsorption depends on sodium reabsorption, which is regulated by aldosterone in the distal tubule and collecting ducts.	a, b, and c. These hormones do not effect chloride reabsorption.
57.	b	Chloride is absorbed in the bowel, mainly the duodenum and jejunum.	a. Chloride absorption does not take place in the stomach.

Question	Correct answer	Correct answer rationale	Incorrect answer rationales
			c and d. Chloride reabsorption does not take place in the liver and kidney.
58.	d	When chloride concentrations drop below 95 mEq/L, bicarbonate reabsorption increased proportionally, causing metabolic alkalosis.	a, b, and c. These are cations, chloride is an anion; a cation must always exchange for a cation in order to maintain electrical neutrality.
59.	c	Potassium is lost via the GI and renal systems. Prolonged or excessive diarrhea can lead to hypokalemia. In the event of hypokalemia, a potassium additive would likely be prescribed.	a. There is no information to indicate the need for this safety measure. b. Antibiotics should be mixed in the appropriate solution; the patient situation provides no information indicating this action. d. There is no information indicating hyperkalemia.
60.	a	Patients experiencing hypokalemia are at risk for digitalis toxicity. Nausea and irregular pulse are signs of digitalis toxicity.	b and c. These refer to concerns regarding hyperkalemia. d. Hypernatremia is not associated with digitalis toxicity.
61.	c	Albumin is a colloid that is used to manipulate fluid shifts among compartments.	a. Whole blood is used to replace blood volume. b. TPN is used for patients who are unable to take in food or fluid. d. Ensure is high caloric nutritional supplement; it is not used to manipulate fluid shifts.
62.	d	Excessive fluid can be lost if breathing and perspiration are at an increased rate for a prolonged period.	a. This is not related to fluid loss. c. This is not an etiology for fluid loss.
63.	c	Lasix will contribute to fluid loss through its action as a diuretic.	a, b, and d. Synthroid (a synthetic thyroid replacement), digoxin (a cardiotonic glycoside), and insulin (a hormone) would not exacerbate fluid volume deficit.
64.	d	As part of the renal regulation of water balance, angiotensin II selectively constricts portions of the arteriole in the nephron.	a, b, and c. These responses do not refer to angiotensin II or any funcions of renal regulation.
65.	a	Approximately 85% to 95% of water absorption takes place in the small intestine. The colon absorbs only 500 to 1000 cc.	b, c, and d. These responses are incorrect.
66.	c	Malabsorption syndrome is associated with hypomagesemia.	a and b. Increased vitamin D intake and diarrhea are associated with hypomagnesemia. d. This response is incorrect.

Question	Correct answer	Correct answer rationale	Incorrect answer rationales
67.	a	Magnesium contributes to vasodilation, not vasoconstriction.	a, c and d. These are all functions of magnesium.
68.	a	The Loop of Henle is responsible for magnesium reabsorption.	b, c, and d. These responses are incorrect.
69.	d	Cardiac arrhythmias are associated with hypermagnesemia.	a, b, and c. Hypertension, tachycardia, and hyperactive reflexes are signs of hypomagnesemia.
70.	a	Green vegetables are high in magnesium.	b, c, and d. These foods are not good sources of magnesium.
71.	b	Decreased cardiac output is a nursing diagnosis associated with isotonic FVD. Other appropriate nursing diagnoses include altered tissue perfusion, potential for injury, and ineffective breathing pattern.	a, c, and d. These diagnoses are not associated with FVD.
72.	b	Weight gain and thirst are symptoms of hypotonic FVE; other symptoms include excretion of dilute urine, non-pitting edema, dysrhythmias, and hyponatremia.	a and d. Poor skin turgor, thirst, hypotension, and pitting edema are signs of hypertonic FVD. c. Interstitial edema and hypertension are signs of isotonic FVE.
73.	b	Potential for decreased cardiac output is a nursing diagnosis associated with hypertonic FVE.	a, c, and d. These nursing diagnoses are not applicable to hypertonic FVE.
74.	c	Isotonic FVD may result from inadequate intake of fluids and electrolytes that can occur secondary to an inability to ingest orally.	a. GI fluid loss through diarrhea is an etiology of hypotonic FVD. b. Insensible water loss during prolonged fever is a cause of hypertonic FVD. d. Impaired thirst regulation is a cause of hypertonic FVD.
75.	c	In third-spacing, fluid is sequestered and is unavailable to the general circulation.	a, c, and d. These responses have no relationship to the third spacing of fluids.
76.	b	Surgical drains will cause a fluid loss, and electrolytes are eliminated along with the fluid.	a. Nasogastric feedings are a source of electrolyte intake, not elimination. c. Immobility does not cause electrolytes to be eliminated. d. Chronic water drinking will change electrolyte levels as a result of dilution, but it does not contribute in any way to electrolyte excretion.
77.	d	In upper gastrointestinal fluid loss, hydrogen and potassium are lost because these electrolytes are present in abundance in the stomach.	a, b, and c. These responses are incorrect because bicarbonate, calcium, and sodium are not abundantly present.

Question	Correct answer	Correct answer rationale	Incorrect answer rationales
78.	a	Bicarbonate is lost in diarrhea because the lower intestinal tract contains fluids rich in bicarbonate.	b. Diuresis is excessive urination that tends to cause a loss of sodium, potassium, and chloride. c. Diaphoresis is excessive sweating that tends to cause a loss of sodium and chloride. d. Vomiting tends to cause a loss of potassium and hydrogen.
79.	b	The renal tubules are the site of electrolyte reabsorption.	a. The glomerulus is the site of electrolyte filtration. c. The bladder is where urine is stored. d. The renal pelvis is where urine travels as it moves from the collecting ducts to the ureter.
80.	b	Electrical neutrality refers to a state in which the same number of positively charged ions and negatively charged ions are present on either side of the membrane.	a. Osmotic activity refers to the attraction of a solute to a solvent. c. There is no such concept as electrical stability in electrolyte balance. d. Sodium–potassium pump refers to the exchange of electrolytes.
81.	a	Body fluids facilitate the transport of nutrients, hormones, proteins, and other molecules.	b. Electrical charges are not transported. c and d. These responses are incorrect.
82.	c	The interstitial space holds 9 L.	b, c, and d. No fluid compartment holds these amounts of fluid.
83.	a	The intracellular compartment holds large amounts of water and proteins. Potassium, lipids, and nucleic acids are also components of the intracellular compartment.	b, c, and d. These are not components of the intracellular compartment.
84.	a	The intracellular compartment holds two-thirds of total body water.	b, c, and d. The extracellular compartment is the interstitial space *plus* the intravascular space. The extracellular compartment accounts for one-third of total body water.
85.	a	The extracellular space contains red blood cells, white blood cells, and platelets in addition to water, electrolytes, and proteins.	b, c, and d. Potassium, lipids, and nucleic acids are intracellular components.
86.	b	The minimum sodium requirement for adults is 2 gm daily. Most adults consume more than this because sodium is abundant in almost all foods.	a. This response is incorrect. c. 4 gm daily would be too high. d. A 1500 calorie weight-loss diet does not give information regarding the salt content.

Question	Correct answer	Correct answer rationale	Incorrect answer rationales
87.	d	Sodium influences the levels of potassium and chloride by exchanging for potassium and attracting chloride.	a. Sodium balance facilitates impulse transmission by participating in the sodium–potassium pump. b. Magnesium is not involved in the exchange or attraction. c. Acid–base balance involves sodium combining with bicarbonate and chloride.
88.	b	The endocrine system secretes aldosterone and ADH to help regulate sodium levels. The pituitary secretes adrenocorticotropin hormone to help regulate sodium.	a and c. These are reproductive hormones. d. ECF is not a hormone; it is the abbreviation for extracellular fluid.
89.	a	The patient is exhibiting signs of hypernatremia and dehydration. The most appropriate nursing intervention is to measure and record intake and output and daily weight.	b. Administration of sodium tablets is not part of the treatment for hypernatremia. Also, the nurse would expect that the IV solutions used for hypernatremia would be hypotonic. c and d. There are no clinical indications for these measures.
90.	b	The patient is exhibiting behavior that could lead to a sodium and water imbalance and is exhibiting signs of hyponatremia. The nurse would check the electrolytes with attention to the sodium level.	a and c. These laboratory results which are not related to the potential problem. d. EEG (electroencephalogram) is a diagnostic test.
91.	b	When recording a patient's intake, the nurse would include all fluids taken by mouth, by nasogastric route, or intravenously. Foods high in fluid content would be included.	a. This response is incorrect because it includes mashed potatoes. c. This response is incorrect because it includes the hamburger and carrots. d. This response is incorrect because it includes the pudding.
92.	a	a. These are altered findings related to intake and output.	b, c, and d. These abnormal findings are related to assessment areas other than intake and output.
93.	a	Temperature elevation results in increased fluid loss through the skin.	b. This response indicates that the fever may be associated with the other symptoms, but it does not provide correct information. c and d. These responses are incorrect.
94.	c	Metabolic acidosis is an acid–base imbalance caused by an increase in metabolic acids. In states in which metabolic acid build-up occurs, metabolic acidosis may occur. Salicylate toxicity causes a build-up of	a and b. These responses indicate that acids are not accumulating. d. Diarrhea causes a loss of bicarbonate through the GI system.

Question	Correct answer	Correct answer rationale	Incorrect answer rationales
		acids, causing metabolic acidosis; aspirin contains salicylate.	
95.	c	Apathy, tetany, carpopedal spasm, low serum potassium, low serum chloride, dizziness, and paresthesia are all assessment findings indicating respiratory alkalosis.	a, b, and d. These responses include some symptoms or laboratory data that are opposite the findings seen in respiratory alkalosis.
96.	b	When monitoring IV therapy, it is important that the nurse ensure that the right solution is infusing at the prescribed rate.	a. This response is incorrect. c. This response does not reflect the IV orders. d. Checking the IV site is only one aspect of the required assessment.
97.	a	Stopping the infusion and removing the IV are actions taken for both local and systemic complications.	b and c. These are not appropriate actions. d. Calling the physician may be appropriate depending on the situation, but not as a first action.
98.	b	Initially after a burn, intracellular potassium is released as cells are destroyed. After 4 to 5 days, potassium may shift from the ECF to the ICF.	a, c, and d. All electrolytes are affected by burns, but potassium shifts represent the most severe.
99.	c	In cirrhosis, aldosterone is not metabolized. This excess presence of aldosterone leads to increased sodium reabsorption and subsequent potassium elimination.	a, b, and d. These choices do not affect sodium and potassium.
100.	b	In SIADH, the antidiuretic hormone is present in excess amounts. This causes too much water absorption, diluting the patient's serum. Water must then be restricted to avoid water intoxication.	a, c, and d. These are not appropriate interventions regarding fluid intake.

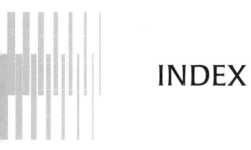

INDEX

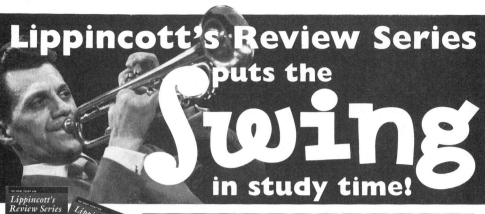
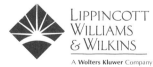

Lippincott's Review Series CD-ROMs provide a convenient way to assess readiness for academic tests and licensure exams. One hundred carefully selected, multiple-choice questions are provided for study and simulated testing. In Study Mode, correct and incorrect feedback with rationale is provided following each question. In Test Mode, questions are scored with feedback available for review at the conclusion of the test

System Requirements

Windows 95 or higher
486/66 Processor or higher
16 MB RAM
6 MB Free Hard Disk Space
256 Colors

Installation

Insert the CD-ROM into your CD-ROM drive.
Click on the **Start** button, and then click **Run.**
At the command line, type **D:\setup.exe.** (Note: The letter D represents the CD-ROM drive. If your drive is designated by a different letter, use your drive letter instead.)
Click **OK.**
Follow the online instructions.

Technical Support

If you experience difficulty viewing the text, it may be the result of the color settings on your system. Should you need assistance or you have any questions regarding the use or content of this CD-ROM, please contact our Technical Support department by telephone at 800-638-3030 or 410-528-4010, by fax at 410-528-4422, or by e-mail at techsupp@wwilkins.com. Technical Support is available from 8:30 am to 5:00 pm (EST), Monday through Friday.

The Trial
of God

The Trial
of God

(AS IT WAS HELD ON FEBRUARY 25, 1649,
IN SHAMGOROD)

**A PLAY
IN THREE ACTS BY**

Elie Wiesel

**Translated by
Marion Wiesel**

SCHOCKEN BOOKS
NEW YORK

Library of Congress Cataloging-in-Publication Data
Wiesel, Elie, 1928–
The trial of God (as it was held on February 25,
1649, in Shamgorod)
Translation of: Le procès de Shamgorod tel qu'il se
deroula le 25 février 1649.
Reprint. Originally published: New York: Random
House, c1979
1. Gezerot tah ve-tat, 1648–1649—Drama.   2. Jews—
Ukraine—Persecutions—Drama.   3. Ukraine—History—1648–
1654—Drama.   I. Title.
PQ2683.I32P7613   1986   842'.914   85-27625
ISBN 0-8052-0809-7

First Schocken edition published in 1986
7 9 8

For Professor Louis Finkelstein

The Trial
of God

CHARACTERS

MENDEL, the oldest, the wisest of them all. In his fifties. Tall, thin, majestic. A dreamer. He is the first minstrel. He knows how to look. And how to listen.

AVRÉMEL, the second minstrel. Melancholy, slightly ironical. A professional entertainer. He knows how to make others laugh, but he himself never laughs. In his forties.

YANKEL, the third minstrel. Noisy, at times coarse. A former coachman, he is restless. Mischievous.

BERISH, the innkeeper. Compared to the other three, he is a giant. Robust, angry. At the first provocation, he could split the table with his fists.

HANNA, his daughter. Mad? Absent. Humiliated, stained. Young, fragile.

MARIA, the servant. Thirty—or less. Tough. Plump but pretty. Outspoken, witty, aggressive.

PRIEST, Russian Orthodox. Short, heavyset, bon vivant. Kind but weak.

SAM, the STRANGER. Intelligent, cynical, extremely courteous. Diabolical. His age? Still young. Neat, almost elegant. Self-controlled.

All are dressed in the style of the seventeenth century. Boots and fur jackets: it is still cold outside. Maria has a black kerchief on her head; the men, fur hats. The priest wears a huge cross on his chest and the traditional robe.

THE SCENE

Somewhere in a lost village, buried in dust and darkness. The time: 1649, after a pogrom. Hate has won; death has triumphed. The rare survivors know that they are alone and abandoned.

An inn, at dusk. A large room with many spots left in darkness. A few tables, chairs. Candles. Empty bottles and glasses here and there. Shadows play threatening games on the walls.

Around a table, three Jewish minstrels order drinks. To forget? To free themselves from a distress that has no name? To celebrate the holiday of Purim whose miracles are told in the Book of Esther?

Purim: the annual day of fools, children and beggars. The carnival of masks. Everybody plays games, everybody gets drunk. Everybody wants to change.

The play should be performed as a tragic farce: a *Purimschpiel* within a *Purimschpiel*.

Its genesis: inside the kingdom of night, I witnessed a strange trial. Three rabbis—all erudite and pious men—decided one winter evening to indict God for allowing his children to be massacred. I remember: I was there, and I felt like crying. But there nobody cried.

ACT ONE

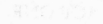

As the curtain rises, MENDEL, AVRÉMEL *and* YANKEL *are sitting at a table.* MARIA *is wiping off the chairs at another.* BERISH *comes in, running; he is annoyed.*

BERISH

A glass, Maria. Hanna will get up any minute, and she'll be thirsty; and there is no glass in her room. I don't understand, Maria—do you? I have glasses everywhere, for everybody, except for Hanna!
(He goes to a table to pick up a clean glass)

MARIA

You're running, running, Master. You're always running. Where to, Master? Where from? Why are you running? (BERISH *stops; he is startled*) Don't you see we've got customers? Hanna is asleep. Leave her alone. When she gets up, I will be there to take care of her, as I always do. But the customers, Master, have you forgotten them? Do I have to do everything, see everything, be everywhere?

BERISH

Be quiet, Maria. Hanna is restless. She'll get up any minute. She'll want her milk. Where have you put the clean glasses?

MARIA

In my pocket. In my bed . . . Don't you see I'm busy? Somebody has to clean up the place—right? (YANKEL *tries to catch their eyes*) You should pay more attention to the customers, Master.

3

BERISH

Don't tell me what to do. You're getting on my nerves. The customers are getting on my nerves. The whole world is getting on my nerves.

MARIA

Then you better get yourself another trade, Master. Better yet, get yourself another world.

BERISH

I'll get myself another helper if you don't stop this.

YANKEL

Leave her alone, innkeeper. Why don't you listen to us instead? We're waiting for you.

BERISH

Who are you?

YANKEL

His Majesty's special emissaries . . . Who do you think we are? Don't you have eyes? We are customers!

BERISH

What do you want?

YANKEL

Service.

BERISH

Service . . .

YANKEL

Does the word sound strange to you? We would like to order drinks.

BERISH

Drinks . . . (*He emerges from his daze*) All that people want is—drinks. (*He places a bottle and three glasses on their table*) One

4

of these days I'm going to close up this place, I promise you that. I'll sell it or burn it to the ground. And I'll get out of here.

MARIA

Right.

BERISH

You don't believe me? I'm telling you, I'll go away.

MARIA

You'll go away, you'll go away. . . . Where would you go?

BERISH

Anywhere. To the end of the world.

MARIA

No farther?

YANKEL
(*Laughs*)

Bravo, woman! Wouldn't you like to join us?

MARIA

Why—are you going to the end of the world too?

YANKEL

No, we have just come from there.

MARIA
(*To* BERISH)

Where *is* the end of the world?

BERISH

I don't know . . . Yes, I do. The end of the world is where you're not.

5

YANKEL
(*To* MARIA)
How do you manage to live under one roof with him?

MARIA
Mind your own business! He's my master. If he feels like
insulting me, let him!

YANKEL
(*Mischievously*)
Wouldn't you like to join us?

AVRÉMEL
The end of the world . . . I remember it well. In my village
there was a small dusty street. An old witch lived in the last
shack. The children were convinced that it was the end of the
world.

BERISH
The end of the world, the end of the world. In my hometown we were told . . . I forget what we were told.

MARIA
Forget it again, Master. You'll feel better.

AVRÉMEL
The witch and her shack. People would be seen entering it
—no one was ever seen leaving it. The children were scared
even to look at it—to look at it from far away.

MARIA
Can't you change the subject?

YANKEL
What's wrong with this one?

MARIA
Change the subject. And change the inn too. You're annoying us.

6

YANKEL

But we've said nothing. We would like to talk to you, innkeeper.

BERISH

I've got nothing to tell you.

YANKEL

How do you know?

AVRÉMEL

What if we asked you not to tell us anything but to listen to us while we tell you something?

BERISH

I'm not interested.

YANKEL

What do you mean, not interested? There must be something that interests you.

BERISH

Right! One thing: to see you get out.

YANKEL

All right, all right. We'll leave. Afterwards.

BERISH

After what?

YANKEL

Have you forgotten that it's Purim tonight? We must celebrate—have you forgotten how to celebrate?

MARIA

Change the subject, *please!*
    (YANKEL *looks at her quizzically*)

7

BERISH

Purim, Passover, Hannuka, it's all the same to me.

AVRÉMEL

Really? It's all the same to you? Then let us tell you. What does one do on Purim? One drinks. Especially when one is thirsty—and we are very thirsty, innkeeper.

YANKEL

Thirsty isn't the word for it.
(BERISH, *exasperated, is about to exit*)

AVRÉMEL

To keep a drink from someone who is thirsty—and on Purim eve, at that—is a sin, innkeeper, a terrible sin!

BERISH

(*Taken aback*)

A sin? Is that what you just said? You shouldn't have said it! Sin is a word I cannot bear to hear! You know why? Because of the sinner. You know who that is? Not I, not you, not even Maria—who knows something about it. It's . . . it's . . .

MARIA

Don't listen to him; he doesn't know what his mouth is saying. It happens to all of us. You are right, tonight is Purim —so we'll drink to that. (*To* BERISH) Do I give them another bottle?

BERISH

Give it to them—but get the money! Make them pay! Is that clear? (*Suddenly he freezes; he has heard* HANNA*'s voice*) A glass, Maria! Quick! Give me a glass of milk, for heaven's sake! Move, woman! Move!
(*He exits hastily.* MARIA *places another bottle on the three minstrels' table*)

8

AVRÉMEL

A strange innkeeper, isn't he?

MARIA

So what! You have your problems, and he has his.

YANKEL

But he *is* strange, admit it. (MARIA *glares at him*) I am not saying this to judge him. If he wants to be strange with his customers, that's his problem—as you just said so eloquently —but that doesn't make him less strange. And besides . . .

MARIA

Besides what? What else?

YANKEL

We could help him; it's our job, you know.

MARIA

Your job is to help strange people?

AVRÉMEL

Our job is to help people. (*Smiles*) Some become strange— later.

MARIA
(*Less aggressively*)

Well, he is not like you or me. But then, who is? Sometimes he keeps quiet for weeks on end; impossible to make him open his mouth—not even to insult me. Then, all of a sudden and without reason, he starts talking, shouting, quarreling: his words just flow and flow—and nothing you do can stop him. You mustn't hold it against him.

YANKEL

Oh, we don't. Why should we? We told you, we are not here to judge him! Besides, we'd rather entertain him.

9

MARIA
(*Laughs*)

Entertain him? You must be joking.
(BERISH *reenters while the three Jews drink and sing a Purim tune*)

BERISH

Not so loud!

YANKEL

We're barely whispering!

BERISH

You're whispering too loud!

YANKEL

Are we in a convent or in mourning? You want us to lament when we are supposed to rejoice? No wonder we're the only customers here; this place is for deaf-mutes with a sore throat.

BERISH

You talk too much.

YANKEL

You want us to stop talking? Nothing could be simpler. (*To* AVRÉMEL) Right?

AVRÉMEL

Right. Pour us another glass. While we drink, we don't talk.

YANKEL
(*To* BERISH)

You are not much of a talker, are you. Is it that you, too, would like another glass? Yes? Have one. It's on us.

BERISH

I'm not thirsty.

10

YANKEL

So what? Must one be thirsty to drink? Do birds fly only when they have someplace to go? They fly because they love freedom and the blue sky. We drink the way they fly.

AVRÉMEL

Listen—do you need reasons? There are reasons. Many reasons. You drink because Purim begins and Yom Kippur ends. Because you're in a good mood—or a bad mood. Because you won—or you lost. Because your daughter is getting married—or can't get married. A Jew who doesn't drink and doesn't know why he isn't drinking—something is wrong with his reasoning, believe me. For a Jew, a day without *yash* is like a love story without love.

MARIA
(*Somber, threatening*)

Did you say love?

AVRÉMEL

What's wrong with love?

MARIA
(*Imitates him*)

What's wrong, what's wrong . . . What isn't? Love was invented as an excuse for everything that goes wrong. You beat up someone and you say, "But it's because I *love* you." You cheat someone and again you say, "But it's because I *love* you." You mention the word love and everything is forgiven. Well, I do not forgive!

AVRÉMEL

A pity you feel that way about the subject.

MARIA

Why?

AVRÉMEL

Because we have got some good numbers on love in our repertoire.

BERISH

I'm not interested.

AVRÉMEL

One song? A shepherd boy singing of his love?

YANKEL

Just one? A shepherd girl dreaming that—

BERISH

I'm not interested.

AVRÉMEL

I guarantee you, you would enjoy it—you really would.

BERISH

I'm not interested, I tell you!

MARIA

How silly can you be! Grown-up men singing love songs about shepherd girls . . .

YANKEL

Why silly? Have you never been in love?

MARIA

Not with a shepherd boy! And I never sang! I am too busy.

AVRÉMEL

Too bad . . .

BERISH

Too bad . . . too bad . . . What do you mean: too bad? Never mind, don't tell me. Just drink up and be quiet!
    (MENDEL *has been listening to this exchange, but seems*

12

remote, absorbed by his own thoughts. When he speaks, the whole mood changes abruptly)

MENDEL

Do you ever pray, innkeeper?

BERISH

Why do you ask? Why do you want to know? What business is it of yours whether I pray or not?

MENDEL

You don't sing, you don't drink, and often you don't talk —so I wanted to know what else you don't do.

BERISH

Well, no. I don't pray.

MENDEL

Don't you know how?

BERISH

I do, but I don't want to.

MENDEL

Any particular reason?

BERISH

That's my business!

MENDEL

Yours alone?

BERISH

Mine alone.

MENDEL

And God? (*Pause*) Where is God in all this, innkeeper?

BERISH
(*Fails to understand*)

God?

MENDEL

Don't you think it's His business as well? Don't you think that whether you pray or not is also His concern?

BERISH
(*Angrily*)

Don't you think He can handle his own affairs? Do you think He needs you to represent Him?

MARIA

I have seen customers fighting among themselves but never with the master. Why don't you change the subject?

YANKEL

You are so wise, Maria. If King Solomon had had a sister, you could have been her.

AVRÉMEL

We have a marvelous song about King Solomon and the Queen of Sheba, would you like us to—

MARIA

Another love story? No, thank you.

YANKEL

Intelligent Maria. Clever Maria. You *are* clever. And careful. Men must be crazy about you.

AVRÉMEL

What a compliment! Doesn't that call for another bottle?

MARIA

Drinks cost money; compliments are free. You have got money?

AVRÉMEL

Don't you trust us? (MARIA *shakes her head*) Poor woman. To live and not to have faith in man is sad, sad—and perhaps sadder than that. How can you love a man if you don't trust him? Answer my question!

MARIA

I have a better one for you: How are you going to pay for all these drinks? I'm warning you—we know how to take care of liars and cheaters and thieves. Don't think for a moment that you'll outsmart us! You won't!

YANKEL

Did I say King Solomon? I was wrong. I really meant Samson. (*He looks at her*) Yes, you remind me of Samson.
(MARIA *wants to reply, but* MENDEL *interrupts her*)

MENDEL

And God in all this, innkeeper? Tell me: Where is God in all this?

BERISH

What do you want from me? Am I His keeper? I resigned from membership in God—I resigned from God. Let Him look for another innkeeper, let Him find another people, let Him push around another Jew—I'm through with Him!

MARIA

Don't you worry, Master. You say things, but God isn't angry. How could He be? He isn't even listening.

YANKEL

Great, Maria! You know what's going on in heaven! Tell us! You're well informed! Are you God's confidante? Tell us! Tell us the truth: are you?

AVRÉMEL

Better yet, He is your confidant! He asks for your advice!

You tell Him what to do and when—and to whom! You even order Him around! Right?

YANKEL

Right! She is protecting her boss by ordering ours around.

AVRÉMEL

Why do you protect him? Why does he need protection? He is hiding things from us, isn't he?

MARIA

The devil with you and your questions!

YANKEL

He's got secrets, right? (*Pause*) So do we.

MARIA

Good for you. Keep them to yourselves.

YANKEL

Don't you want to know what they are? (MARIA *shakes her head*) And you, innkeeper? (BERISH *doesn't bother to acknowledge the question*) Not interested?

AVRÉMEL
(*To* YANKEL)

He thinks our secrets don't concern him. (*To* BERISH) They do, you know . . . You see, we drank your *yash,* we drank well —and we can*not* pay.
(*He bursts out laughing, so does* YANKEL, *but not* MENDEL. BERISH *and* MARIA *look at each other. They're startled at first, but finally join the laughter*)

BERISH

Damn you, jokers! You win—I forgive you. You had your Purim game at my expense. Empty your glasses and go somewhere else. You've stolen enough from me.

MENDEL

Stolen from you? You think we're thieves?

BERISH

No. Just liars.

MENDEL

I protest.

BERISH

Go ahead, protest if you like . . . You show up under false pretenses, you fill your bellies with my drinks, without any intention of paying me . . . So what are you waiting for? Protest!

MENDEL

You misunderstand us, innkeeper. We *can* pay, although we have no money.

BERISH

How? Tell me how.

MENDEL

We'll play for you.

MARIA

There they go again with their love songs . . .

BERISH

You'll play? For me? Have I heard you right?

MENDEL

You haven't guessed, innkeeper? We are *Purimschpieler.* Why do you think we came here? To perform before the Jews of this community. They will pay; not you. For you we shall perform for nothing—in exchange for what you gave us. You see, you were wrong in suspecting us.

17

BERISH
(*Amazed*)

Beautiful! This is beautiful! And funny! (*He is seized with laughter*) Did you hear him? They came to perform! Here! For our Jewish community! (*Sits down*) Did you hear him, Maria? They came to perform a *Purimschpiel* for our Jews—here! Oh, it's funny—it's so terribly, terribly funny!

AVRÉMEL

What's so funny? We haven't begun performing yet, and he's laughing already!

YANKEL
(*To* MARIA)

Has *he* been drinking?
(MENDEL, *too, looks puzzled and questions* MARIA *silently*)

MARIA

Don't you know—don't you *know*—where you are? Is it possible that you don't know?
(*The three performers look at one another, puzzled.* BER-ISH *is still laughing—though now it is inwardly. A spot-light suddenly picks out the* STRANGER, *sitting in a dark corner of the room. He gives a quick smile, and the spot-light goes out*)

MENDEL

Tell us. (*Raises his voice*) I am ordering you to tell us.

MARIA

This is Shamgorod.

YANKEL
(*Freezes*)

No!

AVRÉMEL

You mean this is . . .
18

MENDEL

. . . two years ago. The gravediggers themselves were massa-cred.

AVRÉMEL

We are in Shamgorod . . . ?

MARIA

Near Shamgorod. And you came to play, for the Jews—

YANKEL

We didn't know . . .

MARIA

—the Jews of Shamgorod.

AVRÉMEL

We had no idea . . .

MARIA

That's why you came? To play? Here?

AVRÉMEL

How could we have guessed? We travel a lot—and most villages look alike. All the taverns, all the inns are the same . . .

YANKEL

This morning, as we approached, we thought: This looks like a nice, peaceful place; it must have a good Jewish popula-tion. We'll perform our *Purimschpiel* and make some money— enough to pay for a few hot meals and drinks.
(BERISH *laughs again noisily and stops abruptly*)

MARIA

So—you didn't know.

MENDEL

Sham-go-rod. (*Smiles sadly*) Well, well. We came to perform a *Purimschpiel* in Shamgorod; it had to be Shamgorod!

> (*Now it is his turn to laugh but he cannot;* MENDEL's *inability to laugh is part of his tragedy*)

BERISH
(*Shakes himself*)

So—what are you waiting for? You came to perform? Perform! What are you good at? Well? Sing! Dance—stand on your head! You came to entertain the Jewish community of Shamgorod—so do it! The Jewish population of Shamgorod is waiting!

YANKEL
You are—

BERISH
What's the difference? I am the entire community—the entire population! The last Jewish father alive. Would you refuse the last Jewish father? Let me hear you sing—let me see you make funny faces!

> (BERISH *is excited, annoyed, outraged. He is torn between laughter and despair; he wavers as he seeks ways to avoid one or the other.* MARIA, *aware of his feelings, tries to prevent a catastrophe*)

MARIA
Go, good people, go. You made a mistake—now you know it. You drank and you didn't pay: forget it. Go. Take the road leading into the forest. (*She goes to the window and points*) Walk for an hour and a half or so. You'll find a river. Cross it, and you'll be in another village. There are still some Jewish families left there. Play for them.

BERISH
Yes—go! The sooner the better!

YANKEL
Tonight?

AVRÉMEL

Crossing the river may be dangerous. I cannot swim.

YANKEL

And I'm tired; my bones hurt. And I'm afraid of the forest.

MARIA

It's not too far. Go—you'll rest there.

AVRÉMEL

Can't we stay until tomorrow?

BERISH

No! (*Sarcastically*) Unless you agree to start the performance right away! Well? Go on! Get up! Start the play!

MENDEL
(*Softly*)

How can we? Without an audience?

BERISH

What about me? Am I nothing? And Maria—nothing? We
are nobody? Start!

MENDEL

We cannot, innkeeper. We are not in the mood.

BERISH

I am suddenly in the mood! For a *Purimschpiel!* Yes!

MARIA

Are you sure?

BERISH

Of course I am. Only . . . leave God out of it. You hear me?
I'm warning you!
> (*The three actors get up, put on their masks and move for-
> ward, and form a triangle, facing the audience. At a signal
> from* MENDEL, AVRÉMEL *begins*)

AVRÉMEL

What is life?
What is life?
A road
the child stumbles upon
in his dreams.
What is his dream?
What is his dream?
The hand
of an unknown
in the dark.
What is man?
What is man?
An empty road
for an empty dream.
An empty hand.
What is a drink?
Yes, what is a drink?
The song that fills the road,
and the dream;
the joy that moves the hand
and fills the heart
and gives man
what he never had.

THE THREE
(*pick up the refrain*)

What is a drink?
Yes, what is a drink?
The song that fills the road,
and the dream;
the joy that moves the hand
and fills the heart
and gives man
what he never had.

(*They bow, pull off the masks and start moving back to the table*)

MARIA

You *are* funny. Your joyous songs are sad—sad! I thought that Purim was a happy holiday!

AVRÉMEL

Well—it is!

MARIA

I wouldn't have guessed it—not from your performance! But then, you Jews love to do things upside down. You laugh when you're crying; you cry when you're laughing.

AVRÉMEL

But that's the meaning of Purim, Maria: a story in which everything is upside down. Do you want us to play it for you?

YANKEL

Say yes, woman. For once—say yes!

AVRÉMEL

It's a beautiful story, Maria. Haman plans to kill Jews, and God—

BERISH

Again? This house is off-limits to God, remember?

AVRÉMEL

May we at least recall the miracles?

BERISH

Yes, if you don't give Him credit.

YANKEL

So? Are we playing? I love stories in which Jews remain alive.

23

MARIA

I prefer your other holiday, Yom Kippur, when Jews can't eat—so I eat for all of them.

YANKEL

That's what *you* do on Yom Kippur? Then what do you do when it's *not* Yom Kippur? (*Pause. Grows moody*) But our Yom Kippur lasts all year round.

AVRÉMEL

Stop it, Yankel! Today is Purim! We must rejoice! We're *Purimschpieler!* We must fight sadness, not spread it!

YANKEL

I'm ready. What shall we play if not the story of Purim? How about the story of Joseph? The way he was sold as slave by his own brothers . . . We did it in Zhitomir, remember? People cried—oh, did they cry! They were *so* happy!

BERISH

No! I don't want to cry! And surely not over Joseph! I know all about him! You think I've forgotten his romance with Potiphar's wife? And you want me to weep over *his* tragedy?

YANKEL

Then, let's do the story of Esther.

BERISH

Out of the question! What's *that* story all about? A Jewish beauty who went to bed with an old king whose name is complicated—so complicated that I forgot it—sorry: so complicated that I never even knew it. And they were all there applauding her! Bravo, Esther! You did it! You made it! Now you are a princess! A queen! With an old senile husband who refuses you nothing. Why should I be happy for her?

AVRÉMEL

You're wrong, innkeeper. You insult everybody, but what

24

did Queen Esther do to you? Don't you like her? What don't you like about her?

MENDEL

BERISH

I don't like her story.

MENDEL

What's the matter, innkeeper? Don't you like women?

BERISH

Don't I like women? I love them more than you do! I even love your pretty queen! Let her come to me and you'll see: I'll make her happy. I guarantee it: she'll be happier with me than with her old fool of a husband.

MENDEL
(*Softly*)
And God in all this, innkeeper?

BERISH
(*Mimicking him*)
"And God in all this . . . and God in all this" . . . You're crazy, I swear you are! Can't you talk about anything else?

MENDEL

Do not make fun of God, innkeeper. Do not make fun of God—even if He is making fun of you.

BERISH

If? Did you say if?

MENDEL

It has not been proven yet.

BERISH

What else do you need—what more do you need—as proof? The pogrom of Shamgorod wasn't enough for you?

25

MENDEL

It was and is. More than enough.

BERISH

Then shout it!

MENDEL

I am a beggar. I have learned how to watch, to observe before uttering words that I may regret later. I have learned the art of waiting.

BERISH

I knew how to wait once . . . I waited and waited for redemption, and who do you think came? The redeemer? No: the killers.

MENDEL

And so you choose blasphemy. So be it. But is that an answer? If so, it means there is an answer. I am not sure there is . . .

BERISH

You're too complicated for me. I'm an innkeeper, not a rabbi!

MENDEL

You reject God—I do not. Why not? Because I am intrigued by Him. You see, Berish, I know man; I know what man is capable of. But God in all this?

BERISH

Why don't you ask instead: And Berish in all this? Let me answer you that one: God sought me out and God struck me down. So let Him stay away from me. His company is annoying me. He is unwelcome in my house. And in my life. If He wants to play, let Him play by Himself. If all this is a *Purim-schpiel,* let Him find himself another stage, another theater.

(MENDEL *and* BERISH *look at each other silently.* BERISH

wants to continue but does not: it is useless—God will not
answer. BERISH *is tired; he has said too much*)

MENDEL
(*Smiles*)
I understand your anger, innkeeper. And I like it.

BERISH
Like it or not—who cares? Don't tell me that you share it.

MENDEL
I do not. But I like it anyway. It implies a question—

BERISH
A question? I asked no question!

MENDEL
You did. It is this: in our *Purimschpiel,* who is whose audience? Who is performing for whom?

AVRÉMEL
(*Clears his throat*)
I don't have a question—but I have an answer: Let us perform for you, innkeeper.
(*Again the three actors come forward and form a triangle*)

AVRÉMEL
(*sings*)

The falling leaves
fall for me;
the shining sun
shines for me;
the endless rivers
flow for me.
But I who live
for whom do I live?

27

THE THREE
But I who live
for whom do I live?

AVRÉMEL
The winter nights seem endless
endless for me
but—
(*He is interrupted by the* PRIEST, *who enters, bringing a cold breath of air inside*)

PRIEST
What weather, what weather!

MARIA
(*Sharply*)
Thanks for the information.

PRIEST
Nasty, nasty Maria . . . as always. Why are you so nasty?

MARIA
Why do certain people bring out the nastiness in me?

PRIEST
You inflame their senses, Maria. You incite them to do things they shouldn't even dream about. Why don't you come to confession?

MARIA
I'm scared.

PRIEST
Of what?

MARIA
Temptation. (*Pause*) Yours, Father.

PRIEST
(*Enjoys the joke*)
You can't be fooled, Maria, can you? It's not my fault: the flesh is weak, whereas the devil is not.

MARIA
The devil, the devil . . . You can't do without him; what would he do without you?

PRIEST
I prefer to think of what I could do with you.

MARIA
I see myself as you see me . . . disgusting.

PRIEST
Never mind, Maria, I forgive you—God forgives you. We forgive you the sins we could commit together—if only you would be agreeable.

MARIA
Are you talking about sin or punishment?
(*She leaves him in haste to pour herself a glass of water and him a glass of wine. The* PRIEST *turns his attention to the three Jews and* BERISH, *who, having been interrupted, observe him with an expression of slight annoyance on their faces*)

PRIEST
What are *you* doing here? I haven't seen new Jewish faces here for quite some time.

MENDEL
We are beggars and wandering minstrels.

PRIEST
So you are celebrating tonight? At whose expense?

MENDEL
We are celebrating a Jewish holiday: Purim.

PRIEST

Oh yes, I remember. You are happy because Haman, the great patriot and brave prime minister, was hanged. If you could hang all Christian patriots, that would really be a cause for celebration, right?

MENDEL

Haman was not Christian—if our recollections are correct.

PRIEST

Don't tell me he was Jewish . . . Poor man, how you hated him!

MENDEL

Again—if our recollections are correct—he hated us; he planned to kill us all.

PRIEST

Naturally! What else did you expect? You plotted against him all the time, you had one of your girls seduce his king, so he had to defend himself, didn't he? But you got him in the end, didn't you? You are shrewd; oh yes, Jews always have been. Shrewd and lucky. So you got your man—poor Haman —and nailed him to his cross.

AVRÉMEL

To his what?!

PRIEST

You heard me. Why play the innocent now? Don't you know that Jews killed all their opponents, and always in the same manner. You hate everybody—and then you wonder why you are hated.

MENDEL

We do not hate anybody.

30

PRIEST

Impossible. It wouldn't be natural. How could you not answer hate with hate?

MENDEL

We could—we can.

PRIEST

Impossible. In your place, I would hate the whole world. I would hate heaven and earth. How can you not hate them?

MENDEL

We can.

PRIEST

God doesn't love you, admit it. Tell me: Why doesn't God love you?

MENDEL

I don't know.

MARIA

Neither do you.

PRIEST

Are you taking their side, daughter? You'll burn in hell.

MARIA

Better in hell with them than in paradise with you.

PRIEST

I knew you were nasty, Maria, but not that you were foolish as well. This is the wrong time to show your love for Jews. Things are happening. Shamgorod is agitated because of what occurred in Miropol. A Kotasky child died, and people speak of Jewish malediction and the evil eye. No, daughter, this is not the time for a good Christian to be interested in Jews.

BERISH

Are they starting all over again? Will there never be an end to hate?

PRIEST

As long as there are Jews, they will inspire hate.

BERISH

But except for myself and my daughter, there are no Jews left here!

PRIEST

They can be found elsewhere. In other cities, other villages. Leave it to their enemies; they'll find some to hate. To kill.

BERISH

It's madness, madness!

PRIEST

True, Berish. It is madness and we are helpless. It will disappear when you do, not before.

MENDEL

It will never disappear—not even when the victims are all gone. What would you do if you had no Jews to hate, to vilify, to murder? You don't know? I do. You would begin hating, despising, killing one another. You learn, you practice on us; later you will do it to your own, and then to yourself.

PRIEST

You speak well and without fear. Who are you?

MENDEL

A Jew.

PRIEST

What kind of Jew?

32

MENDEL

Is there more than one kind? In your eyes, all Jews are alike.

PRIEST

You speak without fear—I want to know why.

MENDEL

Beggars learn fast how to vanquish fear.

PRIEST
(*Looks at each of the three*)
I hope this holds true—especially tonight.

BERISH

Why tonight?

MENDEL

I think I understand. (*To the* PRIEST) How bad is it? Be frank with us, please.

PRIEST
(*Bites his lip; then with concern*)
I came here to see you, Berish. I didn't know you had company. I came to warn you. And give you some friendly advice. Go away for a few days, a few weeks. Hide somewhere . . . in the forest perhaps. With friends. Anywhere. Go underground until—until it's over. People are thirsty for Jewish blood, that's all I can tell you . . . (*Takes hold of himself; his expression changes again*) And I am thirsty for some good wine or *yash*. Well, Maria?
(MARIA *serves him.* BERISH *moves closer to the* PRIEST.)

BERISH

Are you serious? Or is it simply your way of scaring us—and getting something in return? Why did you come?

PRIEST

Christian charity, Berish. Pure Christian charity. It still exists, you know. We have known each other for years. I

33

want to help you. Protect you—and your daughter. Can you go away? Stay with a Christian family? I would gladly take you into my home, but it isn't safe: people know of our friendship. How about going to Zhitomir? To Berditchev perhaps?

BERISH

When?

PRIEST

Soon . . . if not sooner. Tomorrow? Tonight? If not . . . if things get bad . . . really bad—we can always use my method.

BERISH

What do you have in mind?

PRIEST

You know, the cross . . .

BERISH

Thank you for that kind of protection!

PRIEST

Do you know one that is more efficient—and less costly?

BERISH

It's like the Angel of Death offering to safeguard the living.

PRIEST

Thank you for the analogy. But then, the Angel of Death has at least one virtue—he is reliable. One can count on him. On whom can you count?

(BERISH *does not reply*)

MARIA
(*Replies for him*)

God.

PRIEST

God?

MARIA

Yes, God. Theirs. Yes—they, too, have a God of their own.
I have faith in Him.

PRIEST

Why shouldn't you, Maria? You are not Jewish. You may
trust the God of the Jews; not they. (*Puts his arm on* BERISH*'s
shoulder*) But you may trust me, innkeeper. I am your friend.
(*To the three Jews*) You, too, I am on your side. Listen to me.
Go away. Right now. And don't say I haven't warned you.
(*The* PRIEST *exits.* MARIA *closes the door behind him*)

MARIA

Don't pay any attention, Master. He's drunk.

BERISH
(*Paces up and down the room*)
I'll kill, Maria. I swear it to you. I swear, this time I'll kill.

MARIA

I could take Hanna.

BERISH

And go where?

MARIA

To Zapritza. My mother's hut is large enough for Hanna
and myself.

BERISH

She stays with me.

MARIA

You come too.

35

BERISH

And they?

MARIA

We could *all* go there.

BERISH

They know about your mother. They would find us in no time.

MARIA

Anyway, we are foolish to pay attention to a drunkard's rambling.

YANKEL

(*Wanting to be reassured*)

Eh, he tried to scare us.

AVRÉMEL

And succeeded very well.

BERISH

(*Still following his vision of horror*)

This time I'll kill, I swear to you, this time I'll kill.

MENDEL

No. (*All look at him, puzzled*) I don't mean you, Berish. Not you alone. I mean all of you. All of us. I said: No. No to fear. What! A few words are enough to stifle our song? Tonight is Purim, and Purim commemorates the end of fear and the beginning of joy.

BERISH

You're a mad, crazy beggar. You're mad.

MARIA

The old man is right! What about—

BERISH

Maria! Are you, too, losing your mind?

MENDEL

Do you have a better solution, innkeeper? No? Then try
ours. Let us proceed. As though the priest had not come. As
though there had not been a pogrom in Shamgorod. As
though killers had no license to kill. Let us celebrate Purim as
our ancestors did.

BERISH

You are mad, crazy beggars. (*Pause*) We are all mad. Purim
is over. For good.

MENDEL

So what! Only madmen know how to pay tribute to Purim!
Purim is for madmen!

MARIA

Long live madness! Long live Purim! Come, I'm pouring
drinks! For everybody, myself included!
(*They drink;* MARIA *serves them*)

YANKEL

Eh, Maria! Are you in love?

MARIA
(*Nastily*)

Is that how you imagine a woman in love? You lack imagination, my poor little minstrel.

AVRÉMEL

How is it to be in love, Maria? What does one feel?

YANKEL

Come, tell us!

MARIA

I'm in a good mood. Why do you want to spoil it? Tonight

37

I want to celebrate with you; tonight I want to forget that I ever was in love—please, friends, leave me alone.

(*They all laugh*)

MENDEL

We have drunk. We have sung. We haven't performed yet. Let's show our gracious host what good actors we really are. What shall we play?

BERISH

Can I choose?

MENDEL

Of course; it's your theater.

MARIA

Long live theater . . . What's theater?

BERISH

When you do something without doing it, when you say something without saying it, while thinking that you did say, and you did do something—anything—that's theater.

MARIA

So—I have made theater! Bravo myself!

AVRÉMEL

What play should we put on?

YANKEL

I've an idea: The unknown master who suffers from being too well known.

AVRÉMEL
(*Shakes his head*)

Too unrealistic.

YANKEL

Then King Solomon and the devil who seized his throne.

AVRÉMEL

Too realistic.

YANKEL

How about—in spite of our host's objections—the story of
Esther? It enables you to drink. A lot . . . Without God, that's
a promise!

MARIA

Good! I'll be the queen.

YANKEL

But you're not Jewish!

MARIA

Nor am I a queen. But who will play the queen? You
perhaps?

YANKEL

Hey, innkeeper, don't you have a daughter?

MARIA

She's a queen, all right, but don't count on her.

AVRÉMEL

I refuse to worship a Jewish queen who is not Jewish!

YANKEL

Then let's play something else. The sacrifice of Isaac? It's
good— It makes you cry!

BERISH

Not me.

YANKEL

Are you against Isaac too? What did *he* do to you?

BERISH

I distrust miracles. They exist only in books, and books say anything.

AVRÉMEL

So do you, innkeeper. You say things . . . Don't you know that certain things may not be said aloud? When I was my community's official jester, I occasionally offended a dignitary, and could, as a direct result, neither eat nor talk except standing. Do you think that God is more indulgent than local dignitaries?

YANKEL

True, how true. *You* could easily be the cause of our misfortunes. You talk, you talk, and suddenly there is a disaster at the door—and it's because you've talked.

MARIA

And the show? And the theater? What's happening to our celebration?

MENDEL
(*Meditating*)

Berish . . . do you know the priest?

BERISH

Eh . . . yes.

MENDEL

Do you know him well?

BERISH

Yes . . . I think so. I know him as one knows a neighbor, a customer—as one knows . . . someone one knows.

MENDEL

What do you think of him?

BERISH

As priest?

MENDEL

As a person.

BERISH

Greedy, wicked like the others. No, it's not true. He is not like the others. Not too brave but not at all wicked.

MENDEL

Should we take him seriously?

BERISH

His sermons?

MENDEL

His warnings.

BERISH
(*Hesitates*)

He drinks a bit, but . . . pogroms should always be taken seriously.

MENDEL

Then a pogrom is possible?

BERISH

A pogrom is always possible.

MENDEL

In Shamgorod? Against whom?

BERISH

Don't you know them? They don't need Jews to unleash a pogrom against Jews.

MENDEL

Maria?

41

I agree. It's possible. Especially since the events took place
. . . The rebellion has driven everybody mad . . . The Ukraini-
ans are angry with the Poles but it is the Jews they're killing
. . . A few words, a few bottles, and the whole village is on
fire. But . . .

MENDEL

But?

MARIA

He is often drunk. He must have remembered the last
pogrom, so he—

YANKEL

Perhaps God will have mercy on us.

BERISH

Starting again?

AVRÉMEL

You don't like it? Don't listen. We need God's mercy—why
not ask for it?

YANKEL

Why not beg for it?

BERISH

Because God is merciless, don't you know that? How long
will you remain His blind slaves? I no longer rely on Him; I'd
rather rely on the drunkenness of the priest. (*Sees the shock on
their faces*) What is it? You don't like the way I speak? How
do you expect me to speak unless you want me to lie? God is
God, and I am only an innkeeper. But He will not prevent me
from letting my anger explode! He will not succeed in stifling
my truth—and neither will you!

MENDEL

What *is* your truth?

42

BERISH

I don't know what it is, but I know that it is an angry truth! Yes, I am boiling with anger! Don't ask me why, you know why! If you don't, I do! But you do know why. You are in Shamgorod, you must know. To mention God's mercy in Shamgorod is an insult. Speak of His cruelty instead. You see what I mean?

MENDEL

I see. Continue.

BERISH

I want to understand why He is giving strength to the killers and nothing but tears and the shame of helplessness to the victims.

MENDEL

So—you don't understand. Neither do I. Is that enough reason to reject Him? Suppose you understood, would you accept?

BERISH

No, I would not.

MENDEL

Why not?

BERISH

Because I would refuse to understand—I would refuse to understand so as not to forgive Him.

MENDEL

Because you have suffered?

BERISH

My suffering has nothing to do with it.

MENDEL

Whose then?

43

BERISH

Whose? (*Changes his tone*) Never mind.

MENDEL

Now *I* want to understand.

BERISH

You won't. Nobody ever will . . .
(*A mood of sadness sets in. Everyone remembers his own experiences*)

MARIA

On my life, I swear on my life, good people, that my master is telling the truth. You will never understand what took place here. What we have seen, nobody should ever be forced to see.

MENDEL

I want to know. (MARIA *shakes her head*) I insist. (*With anger*) I want to know.

BERISH

Look at him! An angry comedian! Since when are *you* angry?

MENDEL
(*Hesitates*)

I don't know . . . No, I do know. It happened in another life. Before I became a minstrel. Before I became a beggar.

BERISH

I was an innkeeper; I still am. And yet I have the impression that since that night I am no longer the same person. That night, life stopped flowing. Nothing matters any more. Nothing exists. Berish is alive, but I am not him. Life goes on, but outside me, away from me.

MENDEL

But life does go on. Isn't that a reason to rejoice? Life continues as before . . .

BERISH

Not as before . . . Before, it was different—I was different. The sap of the earth enriched my own; the blood of the world flowed in my veins. I loved my steady, faithful customers. Occasionally, one or the other—one and the other—misbehaved or refused to pay. Well, my fists were strong enough to teach them a lesson. I was happy and I liked seeing happiness around me. No one left my home or this inn empty-handed. Or with an empty stomach. I loved to give. Why not? I took from the rich and gave to the poor. To glimpse even a fleeting smile on a sad face was for me the most beautiful reward: I had to make an effort to contain my foolish tears. And God in all this? You want to hear the truth? It happened that He would touch me, on the shoulder, as if to remind me: See, Berish—I exist—I, too, exist! Then I would give Him something just to make Him happy: a little prayer for the Sabbath, an act of contrition for Yom Kippur, a good meal for Passover eve. And so, both of us satisfied, we would then go on with our separate daily routines. It's stupid but I can't help it: before, I hardly thought of Him; now I do—and I hate myself for it!

YANKEL

Me—before? I would let the horses gallop away, and I would shout into the wind: I am coming, God of my slain fathers, I am coming to offer you my services. Where do you want me to take you?

AVRÉMEL

I was singing, singing about anything and everything under the sun, and even above—and so was He . . . And we tried to outdo one another.

(*They reminisce nostalgically—except for* MENDEL, *who prefers not to reveal himself*)

MENDEL

And you, Maria?

MARIA

Me? Before your before, I had my own. I discovered love
and the cruelty of love . . . I didn't know that . . . But what
am I doing? Why am I blabbering silly things? You speak of
God, and I— Sometimes, at church, I hear the priest describe
our Lord's suffering—and I wonder whether the Lord isn't
suffering because He must listen to sermons! (*She has an idea*)
Why not accept—or at least consider—his proposal?

BERISH
(*Startled*)

What proposal?

MARIA

The priest's.

BERISH

And go into hiding? You know it would be useless.

MARIA

No, I mean . . . his offer of protection. What would it cost
you? Why not play it safe?

MENDEL

And kneel before the cross?

MARIA

Who would see you? Who would know? You do it one-two-
three and it's over. Do it. Do it for your God or mine. You
know what? Do it for me. To make me feel better.

BERISH

Maria, Maria—why do you talk such nonsense? Would you
want to see us betray our faith?

46

MARIA

I want to see you alive—do you hear me? Alive!

BERISH

You want us to live a lie?

MARIA

Life is not a lie—to live is not a lie! What does it cost you
to pay a silly price for something that is priceless? To bend a
little bit and say a few words while thinking about other
things? What does it cost you to say a few nice words to my
God while silently praying to yours? Your God will forgive
you, I promise you.

MENDEL

Perhaps He will. I will not.

MARIA

I knew it, old man! You are going to give us trouble! Why
did you come here? Why are you harsher than He? Where is
it written that you must die for God? I'm nothing but a simple
peasant woman, I don't know how to read or write. But I
know—yes, I *know*—that life is given by God, I *know* that it
is precious and unique just as God is. God is God: sometimes
He is kind, other times He is not—He's still God! The same
is true of life: sometimes it is sweet, other times it is not—but
life is life and it justifies everything.

BERISH

No, Maria! There are certain things it does not justify.

MARIA

But why, Master? Why? Why make a big thing out of nothing?

MENDEL

To die is nothing?

MARIA
(*Impatiently*)
I'm not speaking about death; I'm speaking about God.

MENDEL
And God is nothing?

MARIA
Don't confuse me—I'm confused already! I didn't say that
God is nothing; on the contrary: He's too much! My God does
not persecute me. Yours does nothing else. Why not play a
trick on Him? Why not turn your back on Him for a day or
a week? Just to teach Him a lesson!

MENDEL
What lesson? That we can go down on our knees?

MARIA
So what! You're on your knees—whisper a few quick sentences—and one-two-three, you're back on your feet!

MENDEL
Wrong, Maria. Once you're on your knees, you can't stand
up straight again.

MARIA
(*Almost hysterically*)
Then make believe! For God's sake, make believe!

MENDEL
That's playing games, Maria! We don't play *such* games!

MARIA
(*Desperately*)
And . . . Hanna? Little Hanna, Master? What about Hanna?
(*A white quasi-transparent silhouette appears at the door.
Frail, she seems to walk on air. They all perceive her presence
at the same time*)

BERISH

Hanna! What are you—

MENDEL

HANNA

Voices—I heard voices. I love to hear voices.

MENDEL
(*With tenderness*)

What do they say?

HANNA

They say that love is possible. And pleasant. That happiness is God's gift to all of his children. They tell me: "Dance." And I dance. They tell me: "Sing." And I dance and I sing. They tell me: "Love." And I love—I love everybody. They tell me: "Live." And I say: "But I *am* alive. Can't you see I am alive?"

MARIA

Come, little girl. Let's go back to sleep.

HANNA

I'd rather stay. You have guests. Do I know them?

MENDEL

No, Hanna. I don't think so.

HANNA

I would like to make your acquaintance, believe me. I am not afraid, I am really not afraid of strangers.

MENDEL

We believe every word.

HANNA

Why should I be afraid? No one has hurt me. Winter nights are quiet here. If some stars are soaked with blood, it is because the sun has penetrated the dark sweet body. Night is screaming, and its screams become stars, don't you see? But

49

that has nothing to do with us, so why should I be afraid of Night? And—

MARIA

You're absolutely right, little girl. There is nothing to be afraid of. And nobody is afraid of anything. Come, let's go to your room.

HANNA

But it isn't polite to leave guests just like that! Please, Maria! (*To* MENDEL) Who are you?

MENDEL

Friends.

HANNA

My father's friends?

MENDEL

Yours too.

BERISH

They're *Purimschpieler.*

HANNA

Really? Oh, I'm so happy. Please, play for me. Sing something—anything! A lullaby? A fairy tale?

YANKEL
(*To* AVRÉMEL)

Well? Go on, sing!

AVRÉMEL

You know the song of the young girl who dreamed and dreamed and never stopped dreaming? Years and years went by and she was still dreaming . . .

HANNA

Oh, I love it! Go on, please!

AVRÉMEL

One night she met a beggar who smiled at her sadly. "I am sorry," said the little girl. "I cannot offer you anything, since I don't own anything; I own nothing, since all this is a dream, only a dream." "It doesn't matter," said the beggar. "I want nothing from you except . . ." "Except what?" asked the little girl. And the beggar answered, "Take me into your dream." And then she awoke.

HANNA

Oh, how beautiful! (*Lowers her voice*) Am I the little girl? Are you in my dream? Am I going to wake up? Will I discover that the beggar has vanished? And you too? (*Laughs*) Do not worry, friends. You will never vanish: I hereby proclaim you immortal!
(*They are all silent and motionless for a moment*)

MARIA

Come, dear. Come with me. You will see our friends again. Tomorrow.
(*The two women exeunt slowly*)

MENDEL
(*Sighs*)

Tomorrow.
(*The silence is heavy*)

YANKEL

I don't know—when I think of tomorrow I remember yesterday. A village, not far from Nemirov. I remember the corpses in the streets and in the courtyards. I remember being told to put them in my carriage and go from nowhere to nowhere. I remember talking to my horse in order not to lose my mind. I remember talking to them as I am talking to myself. And I'm telling them, I'm telling them . . .

AVRÉMEL

The last wedding. The last tune. The last riddle. The guests laugh and weep at the same time. I watch the groom and the bride, I thank heaven for bringing them together. Suddenly —the killers arrive and there is blood everywhere. Everything happens so fast that instinctively I continue to make rhymes; it takes me a long while before I realize that I am trying to entertain the dead.

BERISH

I remember . . . (*Takes hold of himself*) No, I won't tell you what I remember.

YANKEL

Afraid. I remember being afraid. Afraid to go back on the road with another carriage, another horse.

AVRÉMEL

As for me, I was afraid to sing for the dead. Afraid that I could and afraid that I could not . . .

BERISH
(*To* MENDEL)

And you? Aren't you afraid?

MENDEL

Not at all.

BERISH

I don't believe you. You *are*; we all are.

MENDEL

I have seen the limits of truth and the boundaries of man; I have seen farther and looked higher—fear no longer has a hold over me.

BERISH

I don't believe you.

52

MENDEL

I have looked death in the eyes; I have seen God at work.
And I have never turned away.

BERISH

Everybody is afraid. Afraid of suffering or of witnessing
suffering. Afraid of death or of witnessing death.

MENDEL

I am not afraid.

BERISH

Everybody trembles, and you're no exception. The whole
world frightens *me*. Strangers and neighbors, men who are too
drunk or too lucid, too passionate or too indifferent, they all
frighten me. Everything does. Sunshine and darkness. Dawn
and dusk. Streets and cellars. Forests and fields. Clouds and
rainbows. They all help the enemy. Don't protest—you think
as I do. You are also afraid.

MENDEL

I am not afraid.

BERISH

You're lying, you're a liar.

MENDEL

Not I, innkeeper. Not I.

BERISH

"And God in all this?" Have you no fear of God—not even
of God?

MENDEL
(*Hesitates*)
What if I told you that I fear *for* God? You seem to confuse
fear and awe. I am in awe of God, but I do not fear Him.

53

BERISH

I don't believe you. When the whole world is our enemy, when God Himself is on the side of the enemy—when God *is* the enemy, how can one not be afraid? Admit it: you do fear Him. You neither love nor worship Him. All He evokes in you is fear.

MENDEL

Man steals and kills, but it is God you fear?

BERISH

Men and women are being beaten, tortured and killed—how can one *not* be afraid of Him? True, they are victims of men. But the killers kill in His name. Not all? True, but numbers are unimportant. Let one killer kill for His glory, and He is guilty. Every man who suffers or causes suffering, every woman who is raped, every child who is tormented implicates Him. What, you need more? A hundred or a thousand? Listen: either He is responsible or He is not. If He is, let's judge Him; if He is not, let Him stop judging us.

(*The dispute has made them all angry.* MARIA *has returned. She has been listening*)

MARIA

Have you all gone mad? For God's sake, Master, stop talking about God!

MENDEL

We wouldn't mind, Maria. If only He left *us* alone.

BERISH

Right. We shall not let go of Him! (*To the minstrels*) You wanted to put on a play? Do it! But I want to choose the subject. I want a *Din-Toïre!* That's what I want!

MARIA

What's that?

54

YANKEL

That's new; we've never played that.

AVRÉMEL

A *Din-Toïre?* Just like that? On what grounds? Called by whom?

MARIA
(*Annoyed*)

What is it?

YANKEL

A *Din-Toïre* with whom? Against whom?

BERISH

You want to perform in honor of Purim? Good, let's stage a trial! Against whom? Imbeciles, haven't you understood yet? Against the Master of the universe! Against the Supreme Judge! That is the spectacle you shall stage tonight. It is that or nothing. Choose!

MENDEL

You mean a real . . . fake trial?

BERISH

Absolutely!

MENDEL

With God—blessed be His name—as . . . defendant?

BERISH

A trial like any other, except that this time, yes. Yes! With Him as defendant.

YANKEL

And what if the verdict is—

AVRÉMEL

—guilty?

BERISH

So what! It's Purim—on Purim, everything goes! (*Triumphantly*) Well? You agree?

55

(A long silence follows. YANKEL *and* AVRÉMEL *show their reluctance. Not* MENDEL)

BERISH
(Excited)
You agree? Do you?! You have the courage to do my kind of *Purimschpiel?* Tell me! And go to the end of things—and utter words no one has ever uttered before? And ask questions no one has ever dared ask before? And give answers no one has ever had the courage to articulate before? And to accuse the *real* accused? Do you have that kind of courage? Tell me!

MENDEL
(Looks at him intently)
Yes, innkeeper. *(His two friends scrutinize him, startled)* Yes, tonight is Purim, and tomorrow we may be dead. The priest may be right—or wrong; the enemy may win or wait. Let's stage your play, innkeeper. And stage it as free men.

YANKEL
Free to begin—

AVRÉMEL
—and free to conclude?

BERISH
(Jumps up, shouts)
Bravo, my friends! Listen, world! Hear us, mankind! There is going to be a trial!

MENDEL
Tonight we will be free to say everything. To command, to imagine everything—even our impossible victory.
(The spotlight again picks out the STRANGER. *The three wanderers seem to have aged. Only* BERISH *is ecstatic.* MARIA *shakes her head)*

CURTAIN

ACT TWO

The tables and benches have been rearranged to give the impression of a tribunal. The characters perform less than before, now that they are consciously performing specific parts.

YANKEL

I want to have a good time. And wear my mask.

AVRÉMEL

In the courtroom?

YANKEL

Tonight is Purim, yes or no? It's Purim everywhere, yes or no? Can you imagine Purim without masks? I cannot. When I was a coachman, even my poor horse wore a mask on Purim.

AVRÉMEL

But who told you this is the way to celebrate Purim? Your horse?

YANKEL

Please, do not make fun of my horse! My horse brought martyrs to the cemetery! I am not a scholar, I'm a coachman. I taught myself the things I know. And I'm telling you: a Purim without masks is a Purim I don't like.

AVRÉMEL

But we are having a trial!

YANKEL

Let's have it with masks! I love Purim masks!

AVRÉMEL

Because they hide the visible—or the invisible?

YANKEL

Because they are amusing!

AVRÉMEL

What about dignity, Yankel?

YANKEL

What about it? Coachmen have no lessons to learn from jesters!

AVRÉMEL

Don't get angry!

YANKEL

Then stop giving me sermons! I don't like them! You're a judge, I'm a judge: we're equal before . . . before the defendant!

AVRÉMEL

But you don't behave like a judge—you behave like a clown!

MARIA

Oh, I love clowns.

AVRÉMEL

What are we playing tonight: clowns or judges?

YANKEL

What's the difference *what* we play? What's important is that we *play*. And I cannot play if I don't wear a mask!

60

AVRÉMEL

All right, all right! Put it on! Quickly! Go! (YANKEL *obeys*)
If I were to see you in the coachman's seat, I would wonder
who was the coachman and who the horse.

YANKEL

Insulting me again?

AVREMEL

Don't behave as if we were at the market! Please!

YANKEL

What's wrong with being at the market? Why do you make
fun of those who go there? I used to go there often. I loved
it. The sounds, the shouting, the smell. Sometimes I brought
happy people there who returned home unhappy, or the other
way around, simply because they looked where they shouldn't
have. I prefer the market place to the synagogue any day!

AVRÉMEL

Once a coachman, always a coachman.

YANKEL

Now he's against coachmen! Ah, what have we done to
you? Have we stolen your money? Your daughter perhaps?

MARIA
(*To* MENDEL)

Are they playing? (*To the two men*) I, too, like the market
better than the church.

YANKEL

How about coachmen? How do you feel about coachmen,
Maria?

61

MARIA

Men! (*Spits*) They're all alike! I hate men!

MENDEL

(*Authoritatively*)

Enough! (*Pause*) Enough, I said!

YANKEL

Why? Am I not free? You said it yourself: tonight we're all free! Let me do and say what I please! Let me be free tonight.

MENDEL

We are free to play our parts of free men, but not free to act like clowns, Yankel.

YANKEL

Don't clowns have a right to be free?

MENDEL

They do, as clowns. But tonight we are judges. We will speak on behalf of the entire community.

AVRÉMEL

The entire community? What community? There is none in Shamgorod, remember?

MENDEL

Whenever one of us speaks, he speaks for all of us. Even when he is alone, a Jew represents more than himself—he represents a Jewish community, if not the Jewish community.

AVREMEL

(*Pointing at* YANKEL)

That's too complicated for him!

YANKEL

Community, community, I happen to love that word. It makes you warm. But you shouldn't use it too often—not you, Mendel. I like you, I like being with you, but don't think I've forgotten! We coachmen have excellent memories. If I see a face once, it stays with me forever. Well I've seen you before . . . I saw you the day you came to propose to us that we form this company—you belonged to no community then, did you? And when we asked you questions, you were silent. You wished to be alone—and you were. Even with us, you were alone. You never shared your past with us, you never opened up. What do we know about you? That you are a beggar. What were you before you became a beggar? What made you become a beggar? It's impossible to get a word out of you. You and your silences, you and your condescending attitudes, you and your isolation—you have never fooled me. And now you dare to talk about community?

MENDEL

Yes, I do. (*Sighs*) Before, I dared to stay on the sideline. Now I dare to move away from the sideline. And join. And you know what? For the same reasons.

YANKEL

What reasons?

MENDEL

I am not allowed to disclose them to you.

YANKEL

Why not? I want to know. As judge, I have the right to know.

MENDEL
(*To* AVRÉMEL)

You too?

AVRÉMEL

I know. But . . . I don't understand.

MENDEL

That's because of your profession. All your life you tried to entertain. To make people laugh. To do so, you had to learn to know them—not to understand them.

AVRÉMEL

And you?

MENDEL

I—I understood. I sought knowledge and acquired it. To safeguard that knowledge I withdrew from people. And ultimately it was that knowledge that shielded me. But it did not shield others. (*Pause*) What was the difference between the two of us? I didn't try to make people laugh.

MARIA

Try now! Please do!
(MARIA *is ignored by the three judges. She doesn't mind. She keeps busy cleaning glasses, wiping them, putting them away*)

AVRÉMEL

I did. I loved doing that. I loved seeing long, sad faces open up and become warm, good, human. I mean: beautiful; I mean: simple. I used to go from village to village, from one community to another, from one street to another, from synagogue to synagogue, yelling, "Anybody planning a wedding? Anybody contemplating an engagement? . . . No? Really not? . . . Why not? Can I change anyone's mind? . . . Yes? You said yes? Good! Bravo! *Mazel tov!* I am staying. I'll offer a special rate!" Ah, those were the good times . . . Do you know that occasionally people got married simply because I happened to be there? Even after, even during the pogrom, I ran through the streets and market places, through the cemeteries, calling, "Hey, good people, is there no wedding being planned? How about a marriage celebration while I am here?" I made the living cry. As for the dead, I may have made them laugh.

MENDEL
(*Dreaming*)

And God in all this?

64

AVRÉMEL

I don't know. Was He laughing or crying?

BERISH

Speaking of God, how about getting down to business?
(*His reminder brings them back to the present*)

MENDEL

You are right, innkeeper. (*To the others*) Ready?
(YANKEL *and* AVRÉMEL *nod*)

BERISH

One second, please. I have something to say.

MENDEL

We are listening, innkeeper.

BERISH

It's about my part. I want to choose it.

MENDEL

Why? Why you particularly?

BERISH

You mentioned freedom. To be free means to be able to choose.

MENDEL

It's all right with me. Go ahead, choose.

BERISH

Prosecutor. That's what I am going to be. Prosecutor.

MARIA

What's that?

AVREMEL

That's someone nice who has the right to be nasty.

65

BERISH

Tonight I want to be nasty.

MARIA

With whom?

BERISH

With everybody. And more.

MARIA

What will you get from it, Master?

BERISH

Satisfaction. That'll be enough. At last I want to be able to shout, yell, blame, insult, denounce, frighten whomever I please.

MENDEL
(*Consulting his two colleagues*)

I see no objection to that. Congratulations, innkeeper. The court has just appointed you prosecutor. Do you solemnly swear to faithfully and honestly fulfill your duties or . . . don't you?

BERISH

I do, except . . . except for "solemnly."

MENDEL

Ah?

BERISH
(*With a shrug*)

I don't like it.

MARIA

What's that?

BERISH

I don't know, but I don't like it.

66

MENDEL

How about "faithfully"?

BERISH

Yes.

MENDEL

How about "honestly"?

BERISH

Yes again.

MARIA

No!

MENDEL

No, Maria? Why do you say no?

MARIA

That's a word I *do* understand. And I know it's impossible.

MENDEL

Are you suggesting to this court that your master is dishonest?

MARIA

Did I say that? Did I say that my master is not honest? He is! But because he is honest, he cannot say "honestly"! Don't you see?

MENDEL

No, I do not.

MARIA

Really! How can he swear to do something honestly, when he's performing!

MENDEL
(*Smiles*)
All the court expects from him is to perform honestly.

YANKEL
A great day for you, innkeeper!

AVRÉMEL
Mazel tov, mazel tov! Congratulations! With the court's permission, I would like to compose a sonnet in his honor!

YANKEL
Let's celebrate!

MARIA
Again? They'll ruin us!

YANKEL
The occasion calls for drinks!

AVRÉMEL
Yes—the court so orders!

MARIA
The court, what's that?

MENDEL
You don't say "what," you say "who."

MARIA
Have it your way. Who is the court?

MENDEL
We are.

YANKEL
(*To* AVRÉMEL)
Mazel tov.
68

AVRÉMEL
(*To* YANKEL)

I know a song for all occasions:

> *Mazel tov, mazel tov,*
> Luck is with you
> *Mazel tov*
> And so is God
> *Mazel tov.*
> So taste the wine
> And forget the price,
> *Mazel tov . . .*

(MENDEL *silently reprimands him.* AVRÉMEL *bows respectfully*)

MENDEL

With your kind permission, Prosecutor, the court wishes to introduce itself to you. We hope to fulfill our task with courage and wisdom. (*The two judges bow*) And you, Maria, what part appeals to you?

MARIA

None. Unless you need a waitress . . . Oh, how silly of me. I cannot play the waitress, since I am a waitress. Well, I want no part at all.

MENDEL

Everybody plays some part . . .

MARIA

Then I'll play the audience.

AVRÉMEL

Congratulations, Maria! May your star rise and—

YANKEL

Mazel tov! It's simpler. You didn't know you'd get *such* an important part, did you? Ah, if your mother could only be here . . .

69

MARIA

My mother? Why drag her into this?

YANKEL

She would be so proud of you!

MARIA

He is completely crazy!

AVRÉMEL

Never mind, Maria, never mind. It's just an expression we used at home. When a good thing happened, we'd say, "Ah, if my mother could see me now."

MARIA

But she is half blind!

BERISH

(*Impatient*)

Let's forget her mother and remember what we are here for? Let's start!

MENDEL

But someone is missing.

BERISH

Who is that? The defendant? He's used to it.

MENDEL

I didn't mean Him; I meant His attorney.

MARIA

What's that? (*Corrects herself*) Who's that?

MENDEL

That's someone mean who has something nice to say about everybody.

70

BERISH

A flatterer.

MARIA

You mean someone who has the right to lie and flatter other liars?

MENDEL

Well said, Maria. Wouldn't you like to play that part?

MARIA

Oh no! I never lie and I never flatter! I'm being lied to—I'm being flattered: I'm the audience! I'm the masses!

MENDEL

But we *need* an attorney.

BERISH

I don't see why. Since we can do without the defendant, we could do without his attorney.

YANKEL

He is right.

AVRÉMEL

Oh no, sir. We must follow the rules. You may judge someone in his absence but not in the absence of his attorney. We must have a defense attorney in this court.

YANKEL

Obviously.

MENDEL
(*To* BERISH)

Sir?

BERISH

What do you want from me?

MENDEL

You represent authority. The power of the law. It is your duty to find a defense attorney for the defendant.

BERISH

I refuse.

MENDEL

You cannot do that, sir. It's against the rules.

BERISH

Sue me.

MENDEL

Watch your language, sir!

BERISH

Prosecutors watch other people's language! I say whatever I please, how I please. I am free and my freedom is unlimited!

MENDEL

Not so. Only the defendant's is. We are free only to accept or reject the rules of the game—to accept or refuse to play the game.

BERISH

Is that so? Then I won't play. Ladies and gentlemen, the show is over.

MENDEL

Are you threatening the court?

BERISH

Yes, I am. And that's only the beginning! You want to know what I intend to do next? I'll throw you out . . . (*He is ready to add new threats, has second thoughts*) Where do you expect me to get hold of a defense attorney? First, I don't know any. Second, there is none in Shamgorod. Third, even if there were, he wouldn't be Jewish. Lastly, I've nothing else to say.

(The prosecutor and the judges gaze at one another. Where are they going to go from here?)

AVRÉMEL

I want to say something.

YANKEL

Is it urgent?

AVRÉMEL

Always.

MENDEL

Only if it is related to the present debate.

AVREMEL

It is. The prosecutor urgently needs to be taught some manners.

BERISH

I protest! (MENDEL *looks quizzically at* AVRÉMEL) It's unheard of!

AVREMEL

May I continue?

MENDEL

Please. But, dear colleague, remember that as judges we are committed not to offend anyone.

AVREMEL

As judges, it's our duty to protect the dignity of this court. Therefore I'm asking the prosecutor not to scratch his beard when appearing before us: this is not a tavern, if I may say the obvious. Also, when addressing the court, Prosecutor, you're bound to show us consideration and respect, even though you are longing inwardly to break our bones. Yell until tomorrow, but not at us. Also, and in the same order of ideas, I—and we

73

—would appreciate it if you would begin or end, or both, every sentence with the customary expression: Your Honor!

BERISH
(*Doesn't understand*)

Your—what?

AVRÉMEL

Your Honor.

MARIA

What's that? Or is it, who's that?

BERISH

Tell me, are you *completely* insane or only mostly?

AVRÉMEL

He's insulted the court! I demand he be indicted for contempt!

BERISH

Maybe we need a doctor, not an attorney!

MARIA

We had a doctor. He was killed.

MENDEL

Prosecutor, please try to understand that my colleague's statement is not aimed at you personally.

BERISH

No? Then why did he talk to me?

MENDEL

He talked to you but he didn't mean to offend you.

BERISH

Whom then?

74

MENDEL

No one. All he meant to say is that there are certain customs
and forms we must all adhere to.

BERISH

Not I! I don't know these customs and do not wish to know
them!

MENDEL

What are you afraid of, Prosecutor? Listen, at home they
called you Berish, right? (BERISH *nods*) Your customers call
you innkeeper, right? In the synagogue they call you Reb
Dov-Baer ben . . .

BERISH

Yaakov.

MENDEL

Yaakov. See? We address one another differently according
to the place and to the circumstances that brought us together.
So here, in the courtroom, you address us as Your Honor,
that's all.

BERISH

And how will you address me?

MENDEL

Very respectfully, sir.

BERISH
(*Surmounts his hesitation*)
All right, if you say so . . . Your Honor.

MENDEL

Good! Excellent! You see? You learn fast! I compliment
you on your amazing progress! Except we still don't have an
attorney.

BERISH

To hell with him . . . Your Honor.
(YANKEL *and* AVRÉMEL *seem offended, but not* MENDEL)

MENDEL

We need an attorney; we cannot start our proceedings without one. You do understand that, don't you, sir?

BERISH

But there is no one to serve as attorney, don't *you* understand that? (*Stops to reflect*) Your Honor, must the attorney be
a man?

MENDEL

Not necessarily.

BERISH

(*Moves toward* MARIA)

Maria!

MARIA

Oh no, Master. I'm the audience, remember? The people.
And the people are more important than anyone. More important than attorneys. More important than prosecutors. And
judges. You can do without Your Honor, but not without the
people.

BERISH

What nonsense! You are not the people, you are you.

MARIA

Sorry, Master. Don't count on me.

BERISH

Do it for me.

MARIA

Sorry, Master. Don't get angry at the people; the people
won't like it. The people want you to be gentle and tender—

76

BERISH

I'll kill you, you witch!

MARIA

Why? The people can say anything they please—

MENDEL

Right. Under one condition: that they do not say it.

BERISH

I'll kill her if she doesn't help me out, I'll kill her.

MARIA

Don't get angry, Master. I am not an attorney—I don't even know what an attorney looks like. I don't even know what he does, what he says. Must he believe in law and justice to defend them—or the opposite? You see, Master, I'm too ignorant. . . . And also, I'm not even Jewish!

YANKEL

Hmmm.

MENDEL

Is my illustrious colleague asking for the floor?

YANKEL

(*Clears his throat*)

My Honor wishes to tell Your Honor something very important.

MENDEL

The court will listen to you eagerly and sympathetically.

YANKEL

When Srulik the butcher needed my coach to bring him to Nadvorno, I told him that my horse was sick. So he brought his own.

ALL

So?

YANKEL

So I wonder whether we—the tribunal—couldn't ask the defendant to bring His own attorney. Or to be His own attorney.

(*Laughter*)

BERISH

(*Sneers*)

Ask Him, why not? What are you waiting for? (*He becomes serious*) Never mind. There are two possibilities: either we play without attorney or—we don't play at all!

ALL

Not at all! What a shame . . .

BERISH

Well, if you insist on the attorney, there is nothing we can do—except abandon the whole idea. I'll go to bed and you—out!

(*The threat is real, and all sense it. Their only chance to stay is to stage the play*)

ALL

No, no! Impossible!

MENDEL

Do you have a friend in the neighborhood?

BERISH

No. I told you, there are no more Jews around.

MENDEL

You, Maria? Can you think of anyone who might do?

78

MARIA
(*Hesitates*)

No . . . No.

BERISH
(*Nastily*)

Oh, she had somebody. But he left. (*Moves closer to* MARIA)
Look, she's blushing!

MARIA

Leave me alone, Master.

BERISH

Why are you blushing? He was a nice man. Strong and
handsome. Look! She's blushing! (*Pause*) He seduced you,
didn't he?

MARIA
(*Troubled, angry*)

Please, Master. Why do you want to hurt me?

BERISH

You spent the whole night with him, didn't you? You think
I didn't see you? I saw you in his arms . . . He left you. Why
did he leave you?

MARIA

This is not the time, Master . . . Please!

BERISH

What was his name?

MARIA

His name? . . . His name was—Sam.

BERISH

Sam—what?

MARIA

Just Sam.

BERISH

No last name?

MARIA

Only Sam.

BERISH

Lack of manners! He didn't introduce himself to you? And you let him take you? A stranger? (*To the court*) He appeared shortly before the pogrom, spent the night here and left in the morning. (*Pause*) He was a Jew, he spoke Yiddish to me. To her he spoke . . . What did he speak to you, Maria? You didn't speak, is that it?

MARIA

Master, I beg of you. Stop it.

BERISH

What did he promise you? What did he offer you? He would've been perfect for the job . . . for any job, I might say.

MARIA
(*Close to tears*)
Please, please! Stop talking about him!

BERISH

How *did* he seduce you? What did he tell you? What did he promise you?

MARIA

You're cruel, Master! God will punish you . . . He already has!

MENDEL

Have you seen him since? No? Do you know his where-
abouts?

MARIA

I beg you, old man, stop torturing me!

BERISH

But what about the damn attorney?! Because of him we'll
be deprived of a trial! (*To* MENDEL) Is there no way of getting
around the difficulty? How about . . . bribery? I've heard of
judges being bought, you know . . .

MENDEL

Wait. (*All stare at him*) Actually, in the ancient Jewish tradition, trials were conducted without defense attorneys—

BERISH

(*Exuberant*)

Good heavens, why didn't you remember that sooner?

MENDEL

—and without prosecutors.

BERISH

(*Shocked*)

You want to get rid of me already? Are you asking for my
resignation? If you oust me, I'll oust you. Just try it! With or
without Your Honor, you'll be in the street one-two-three!

MENDEL

Don't get excited, innkeeper! You're the best prosecutor
we've got. You see, in ancient times, when innkeepers were
innkeepers, judges were required to be able to handle both
the prosecution and the defense of an accused. But now, everything has changed, the legal system itself has changed. We
may therefore adapt it to our situation. Since we already have
a prosecutor, we will ask a member of this court to serve as
both judge and attorney for the defense.

BERISH

You are a genius! And so I offer you ten free meals beginning tomorrow—

YANKEL

Bribery, this is bribery!

BERISH

—and ten for you too.

YANKEL

Yes, as I was saying, this might appear to be bribery. But it isn't! For if it were, who would prosecute the prosecutor?

AVRÉMEL

Let's vote.

MENDEL

A suggestion has been made to appoint a member of this tribunal attorney for the accused, whose absence ought not be misinterpreted. Who is in favor?

YANKEL

Couldn't we vote *after* the meal? (*He looks at* MENDEL *questioningly*) All right, I'm for it! And what about you, jester?

AVRÉMEL

I am hungrier than you.

MARIA

Ten meals . . . multiplied by three . . .

MENDEL

The audience is requested to keep its comments to itself.

MARIA

You mean you all may speak but I may not?

82

YANKEL

This woman keeps on interrupting our proceedings; I demand she be jailed and punished.

BERISH
(*To* MARIA)

Offer them twenty free meals, hurry!

MARIA

Twenty? Why twenty? You want them to stay a whole year?

MENDEL

Woman, you are under arrest.

MARIA

All right, twenty.

MENDEL

You're under arrest.

MARIA

I said twenty. That's not enough? All right—thirty.

MENDEL

Never mind. Just apologize to the court.

MARIA

I have the honor to tell Your Honor—and Yours—and Yours—that I am sorry for having doubted your honor.

MENDEL

We may proceed. (*To* AVRÉMEL *and* YANKEL) Who volunteers to serve as lawyer for the accused?

YANKEL

I know one thing—and I know it well; I know who will not volunteer: I.

MENDEL

You refuse?

YANKEL

I didn't say that. All I said is that I *know* who will not volunteer.

MENDEL

That means you refuse.

YANKEL

I speak of what I know; you speak of what you do.

MENDEL

But why, Yankel? To defend the Creator of all things, the Judge of all mankind, the King of Kings—is there a greater honor than that?

YANKEL

Thank you for bringing me customers. As a passenger, I would take Him: He doesn't take much room. Here it's different. First, I don't know what and if He'll pay. You'll tell me: could you be sure that He'd pay for his coach fare? No, I couldn't. But it's not the same thing. He'd sit in the coach and the horses would do the pulling; in court, I'd be the horse. So why do it at all? Second, and that's worse: Suppose I lose the case? No, it's not for me. Let someone else take this case.

MENDEL

And you, Avrémel?

AVRÉMEL

Yes, of course—I mean: no, of course not.

MENDEL

But in a way, it's your profession, isn't it? You were a minstrel. You know your way around with words. Make up a few for Him—why not?

84

AVRÉMEL

Such a client deserves a better attorney. I would only shame
Him. With me as lawyer, He risks finding himself in hell
. . . Oh, what am I saying? I hope He didn't hear me. If He
did, I will be the one who needs to be defended.

BERISH
(*Amused*)
There is one more candidate left. (*Pause*) You.

MENDEL

As president of this court, I declare that the president has
not been and *is* not a candidate.

BERISH

Why not?

MENDEL

As president, I don't have to tell you.

BERISH

I have the right to know.

MENDEL

And I have the right to deny you your right.

YANKEL

The prosecutor wants an explanation. So do we! We ex-
plained. Why don't you?

MENDEL

Because.

AVRÉMEL

That's not an answer?

MENDEL

Nothing is.

BERISH

I protest!

MENDEL

Good for you.

YANKEL

We all protest.

MENDEL

Good for you, too.

BERISH

Listen, beggar of my heart, you deny me the right to know, and this is unfair. What is the purpose of this trial? We know perfectly well that the outcome won't change anything: the dead will not rise from their graves. We judge because we wish to know. To understand. In order to understand others, I must understand you too! Speak up, for heaven's sake!

MENDEL

As president, I choose when to speak and when to keep quiet. Now I have chosen not to speak.

BERISH

I object!

MENDEL

Objection overruled.

MARIA

The people protest!

MENDEL

I shall have the courtroom evacuated if you persist!

MARIA

I protest—the people protest against your not letting me protest!

BERISH

Objection!

MARIA

More objections!

YANKEL

Booo!
> (*They shout and shout. Then, spent, they become motionless, silent*)

MENDEL

You forget why we have gathered here tonight? (*Pause*) The question remains a question: Is there no one here—or anywhere—to plead the cause of the Almighty King of the universe?
> (MENDEL *has spoken with nostalgia. Melancholy sets in*)

AVRÉMEL

Poor, poor King of Kings.

YANKEL

Feel sorry for Him? Already?

BERISH

We're heading in the wrong direction! We're here not to pity Him but to judge Him!

AVRÉMEL

Poor King who needs His servants' pity.

BERISH

He needs it? He won't get it! Not from me! He had no pity for me, why should I have for Him?

87

MENDEL

I—who? Berish the innkeeper or Berish the prosecutor?

BERISH

Berish is Berish.

MENDEL

But who is Berish? An innkeeper who plays the part of prosecutor, or a prosecutor who happens to be innkeeper?

BERISH

Don't confuse me. I am I. Isn't that enough for you?

MENDEL

Anyone can say "I."

BERISH

You confuse me. I protest.

YANKEL

I—who?

BERISH

I—Berish. And I'm fed up with you! I'm an honest man, I've never stolen, I've never cheated! I've never humiliated anyone! I have done only good, not He. He has done me nothing but harm. And now, now you want me to feel sorry for Him? Where was He when . . . (*Catches himself and tries to sound calm*) I forgot that we are playing—maybe He, too, is playing. (*To* MENDEL) Who are you when you're not playing? Tell me. I want to know.

MENDEL

Why?

BERISH

Say that I love to know the truth. About me—and you. And Him. And everyone else. I know what we're about to play but not with whom I'm about to play. Tell me.

88

YANKEL

Don't waste your energy on him; you'll get nowhere. He is a rich beggar; he has a secret treasure; his treasure is his secret.

BERISH

And you are not even curious to find out?

YANKEL

Questions are like trips: we must know when to stop. Coachmen have to think of their passengers. And the horses.

BERISH

Let them drop dead.

YANKEL

Who? The passengers?

BERISH

The horses.

YANKEL

What have they done to you?

BERISH

Nothing, nothing. *You* are annoying me, not they. You're all getting on my nerves! A nice Purim you've arranged for me!

MENDEL

You are asking too many questions, innkeeper. Purim is not the time for that. Purim is the story of Esther, and Esther means secrecy. Everything remains hidden, and it's not up to you to reveal it. You, as prosecutor, must bend before the law.

BERISH

I'm ready to bend before the law, but I insist on understanding it! I want to know what is happening and why!

MENDEL

So do we, innkeeper.

BERISH

But you are not I. I want to know why human beings turn
into beasts. So do you. But you haven't seen them. I want to
know how good family men can slaughter children and crush
old people.

MENDEL

So do we, innkeeper.
(BERISH *yields. His mood changes*)

BERISH

What strange birds you are. I don't know who you are, but
I know that you are strange. Where do you come from? Who
sent you? Who are you?

YANKEL

His curiosity will do him in, I am sure of that.

AVREMEL

He *is* going too far.

YANKEL

He is drunk, after all.

BERISH

Drunk? Me? Too easy. Why do you say that I am drunk?
Because I want to know who you are? Strangers make me feel
uneasy. They come and go, and I stay behind like an imbecile.
You'll tell me, what about the defendant? Isn't He a stranger
too? Yes, He is, but not really. I know Him, oh yes, I know
Him. In my own way, I know Him, all right. He is like a
customer; you don't need to know customers: you sell them
food and drinks; they go and I keep their money. But you are
not customers. You can't even pay your bill—you are something else and I want to know what.

Who.

You're right, witch. Who, what, it's all the same. They're making fun of us.

(MENDEL *examines him closely and begins to speak to him in the manner of a teacher talking to pupils. Gradually his voice rises and gains tension and anger*)

MENDEL

You are funny, Berish. The innkeeper yearns for justice, and the prosecutor will settle for knowledge. Have you forgotten what tradition has taught us? We must drink *Ad d'lo yada*—we are bound by law to drink and drink, and drink more, until we are unable to distinguish between good and evil, between Mordechai the Just and the wicked Haman, between light and shadow, life and death. Purim signifies absence of knowledge, refusal of knowledge. Are you going to change tradition? Establish a new one? On whose authority? (BERISH *makes a movement*, MENDEL *notices it*) Are you going to threaten once again to send us out into the street? Stop threatening! It won't work! You are no longer free to withdraw! Once the trial has begun, it has to be brought to a conclusion!

BERISH
(*Retreats*)
You are touchy, aren't you? All I wanted—

MENDEL
All you wanted was—what? What did you want? To begin at the end? To force us to prejudge the case? Enough of your diversionary tactics! We are dealing here with a unique case with unprecedented implications! Our judgment may prove useless but not meaningless! You want to know who we are? We are members of a rare tribunal whose authority derives from its own sense of justice and perhaps humor. You want to know more, and go

to the end of all worlds; you want to tear off all that covers certain words, break the vessels of—

(*His violent tirade is interrupted by the* PRIEST*'s re-entrance. Sudden silence. Renewed fear*)

PRIEST

Maria, Maria, here I am again, you see? I need you. I need to save your soul—even if you reject me. Come, daughter. Come, give me another drink. I need strength to take care of your salvation. (*At* BERISH*'s signal,* MARIA *hands him a drink*) Yes . . . (*He addresses* BERISH *and the three Jews*) and of yours as well . . . You are in great danger, believe me. Heed my warning.

MARIA

You're repeating yourself, Father.

PRIEST

So does our Father in Heaven, Maria. So does He. How many times has He been repeating to us the teaching of His love? But you refuse to love Him, as you refuse to love me. Is it that you are unable to love altogether, Maria? It's because of your sinful adventure with the Stranger; I swear that it's that night that you lost your soul . . . Remember that night, Maria? I do. You were together, I saw you . . .

MARIA

You dirty pig—you Peeping Tom—and that claims to be God's servant!

PRIEST

You sinned, Maria. Remember, Maria, you let yourself be seduced by the Stranger, and punishment struck soon after, remember?

MARIA

It didn't strike me! It struck those who had not sinned! You better look for a better example!

PRIEST

I am not looking for any, not now, daughter. You think I came back to preach? I came to help you. I want to help you. Don't ask me why. Perhaps it's because I can't forget the last time . . . It happened here, Maria. I was present. And you, too. And Berish. And Hanna. And—

MARIA

Enough, Father!

PRIEST

I don't want it to happen again. I'm responsible for my flock . . . I want to prevent further bloodshed. And there will be bloodshed, believe me. There is hate. Hate leads to blood-shed. I came to you in the name of heavenly love.

YANKEL
(*To* AVRÉMEL)

How about inviting him to play in the show?

BERISH
(*To the* PRIEST)

We're grateful. Touched by your kindness. But we're busy. Come back another day, another evening.

PRIEST

Another day? Will there be another day?

PRIEST

Some people always think they have time. They're on the edge of the abyss and don't want see; they're singed by the flames and don't realize that they're already in hell.

MARIA

Hell? Is he talking about hell? Good. For a moment I was afraid he was making sense.

PRIEST

I am talking about hell because . . . because I always do. It's a matter of habit. And it's easier. But you're wrong in not listening . . .

Another time. Do come back another time. Hell will wait, I promise you.

But it's late, innkeeper. Much later than you think.

Right you are! Much later! So go home, go back to bed.

Don't worry over me; I risk nothing. You do. You risk a lot. I told you, didn't I? Go away. Take your family, your friends, and go into hiding. In the woods. Anywhere. If you've nowhere to go, come to my house—the House of the Lord. (*Pause, then more gently*) You'll be in relative safety. It's safer than here . . . Oh, I've not come back to convert you. Be damned if that's your desire. But I want to protect you from the mob. You must believe me, Berish, you must.

You *have* become charitable all of a sudden! What has come over you?

The mob is mine, Berish. I'm in charge of their souls. I don't want to see them commit murder again. I saw enough the last time.

Is the danger that imminent?

Could anything happen *tonight?*

94

PRIEST

It's possible. Everything is possible. I've got a good nose.
I can smell bloodshed. I feel the mob getting ready.

MARIA

You have a nose, yes? And what about the last time? Where
was your nose then? Why didn't you warn us the last time?
(*Her hate is tangible, visible*)

BERISH

Maria!

PRIEST

You're right, Maria. I should have; I didn't. But then, I
tried to save you, Berish, didn't I? I did my best, didn't I?

BERISH

Yes, you did. You offered us the protection of the cross.

PRIEST

That was your best chance, Berish! If you had accepted,
your sons and their mother might still be alive!

BERISH

Enough! Not another word!

PRIEST

You're angry and I know why. We were friends and I
couldn't protect your family. But I am still your friend, more
than ever. You must listen to me. You must believe me!

MENDEL

You really think it could happen tonight?!

PRIEST

Yes.

MENDEL

But you're not sure?

PRIEST

No.

MENDEL

Then we will think about it.

PRIEST

When?

MENDEL

After the play.

PRIEST

After what?

MENDEL

After the play.

PRIEST

What? A mob is getting ready—knives are being sharpened —and you're acting?

MENDEL

Outside, Haman's mob is getting ready, while inside, the Jews went on with their prayers; that was their idea of theater.

PRIEST

May I stay and watch?

MENDEL

No, you may not.

PRIEST

Why not? Are you going to say bad things about me or my people?

MENDEL

No, neither about you nor about your people.

96

PRIEST

What is the play about?

MENDEL

We don't know yet. It's going to be an improvisation.

PRIEST

Looking for ideas? How about staging a conversion? No?
A pity. What a pity.

MENDEL

Thank you for the suggestion, but—

PRIEST

I understand, I understand. (*Walks to the exit, stops*) No, I
do not understand. You, Berish—were you ever known for
your piety? Were you seen more often with drunkards or with
rabbis? Then tell me: Why this sudden loyalty to your God—
why?

MENDEL

Our relations with God are our business—ours alone.

MARIA

Is *he* preaching *here?* To you, Master? Where does he think
he is? In church?

MENDEL

There is the people of Israel and there is the God of Israel:
Let no one interfere in their affairs!

PRIEST

So, you forbid me to help you, to save you, is that it? All
right, then. Go and hand yourselves over to the sword. You'll
get what you deserve. Amen. (*Pause*) God doesn't love you
anymore, admit it. He has turned His face away from you.
Why don't you see the truth as it is? He is fed up with you.
He is disgusted with you . . .

97

MARIA

Wicked drunkard!

BERISH
(*To the* PRIEST)
Look who's talking! If someone is disgusting, it's you!

PRIEST

God, the God of your fathers, has given up on you. That's why He handed you over to us—the servants of Christ, His Son. From now on, we shall be your masters, your rulers; we shall be your God. Why would we be invested with such powers if it were not for God, who entrusted us with a mission to you, His rebellious children? It is the will of God that we, Christians, shall be your God.

MENDEL

That you are God's whip, that is quite possible. But don't be so proud of it! God is closer to the Just struck by the whip than to the whip. God may punish the Just whom He loves, but despise the instrument of punishment; He throws it in the garbage, whereas the Just will find his way to the sanctuary.

PRIEST

Don't go too far! You have just thrown into the garbage my Lord! He is the Son of God!

MENDEL

We all are.

PRIEST

You were once. He disowned you.

MENDEL

Are you certain of that? How can you be so sure? Because we suffer? Between the man who suffers and the one who makes him suffer, whom do you think God prefers? Between those who kill in His name and those who die for Him, who, in your judgment, is closer to Him?

PRIEST

Now you speak of Christ as an assassin! How dare you!

MENDEL

Wrong—you haven't been listening. I speak not of Christ but of those who betray Him. They invoke His teaching to justify their murderous deeds. His true disciples would behave differently; there are no more around. There are no more Christians in this Christian land.

PRIEST

(*Calm again*)

Is it His fault? Why blame Him? If what you say is true, then feel sorry for Him. If Christ is alone and abandoned—then it's up to you, His brethren, to comfort Him.

MENDEL

We will, Priest. One day we will.

PRIEST

One day, one day—you Jews love to see far ahead. Another day, another day. Not now, later. Then it's too late . . . Will you remember that I warned you?

(*He exits slowly. All the actors follow him with their eyes. He opens the door. The wind outside makes the candles flicker*)

MENDEL

What happened the last time, innkeeper?

BERISH

Forget it. I'm not going to tell you.

MENDEL

We would like to know.

BERISH

Too bad. Did you answer my questions? Why should I answer yours?

MENDEL

Maria . . .

BERISH

She won't answer you either!

MENDEL

Maria, perhaps you ought to go to the window from time
to time. Keep watching. One never knows.

MARIA

The priest talks a lot, that's all.
  (*She would like to reassure her friends. They now feel the
  danger.* BERISH *also knows that there is no way to avoid
  it*)

BERISH

Can we return to the play?

MENDEL

No.

BERISH

Why not?

MENDEL

No defense attorney.

YANKEL

Don't count on me.

AVRÉMEL

Or me.

MARIA

You are all funny. When you want to accuse, you are here,
ready to judge and pass sentence. But when you are asked to
defend, you turn around and start running.

100

MENDEL

What about Hanna?

BERISH

What do you have in mind?

MENDEL

She could play the defense attorney.

BERISH

She's sick. Let her be. You don't ask a sick person to play a sick person.

MARIA

Poor, poor Hanna. Does she realize what's happened? What will happen?

BERISH
(*To the three judges*)

How about flipping a coin? Let fate decide.

YANKEL

I don't like it, but—

AVRÉMEL

I don't like it without but.

MENDEL

I could appoint one of you.

YANKEL

You can force a horse to run but not to neigh.

AVRÉMEL

You can force the coachman.

YANKEL

You cannot. But you can force a jester to sing.

AVRÉMEL

No. You cannot.

MENDEL

Then it's a deadlock.

MARIA

Who's that?

MENDEL

We are at a point from which it is impossible to proceed. We are standing still.

MARIA

And waiting?

MENDEL

And giving up.

MARIA

The people says no.

YANKEL

Let the people keep quiet and say no later.

AVRÉMEL

Perhaps it's for the best. If the priest is right, then we could use the time for more urgent things. For instance: we could run.

YANKEL

And run fast!

MARIA

The people has changed its mind; I say yes. Let's start looking. Packing. Move out. The priest is drunk, but I don't have too much faith in his drunkenness.

AVRÉMEL

So—we stop the play? And run?

YANKEL

We stop the play. Goodbye, Judge. Good evening, Minstrel. It'll be nice to meet you again.

MARIA

Let's go to the forest; we could at least lie down and rest. And gather some strength for tomorrow.
(YANKEL *and* AVRÉMEL *get up.* MENDEL *remains seated.* BERISH *sizes them all up and explodes*)

BERISH

All right, go! Go, all of you! Go to bed! Go to sleep! Have pleasant dreams! Cowards, imbeciles! Even to play against Him frightens you! Scared to open your mouths! The attorney? A convenient pretext. The rules? An excuse. In truth, you didn't dare continue! In truth, you were planning to stop in the middle from the very beginning! You were waiting for the right moment to run away with your heads lowered and your hearts full of contrition! I know your kind. Go away! Out of here, out of my sight! I don't need you! I'll play without you. I'll yell for truth all by myself! I'll howl words that have been howling inside me and through me! I'll tear off all the masks of Him whose face is hidden! With or without an attorney present, Your Honor, the trial will take place!

YANKEL

But, innkeeper, it's irregular!

AVRÉMEL

If there is a prosecutor, there must be a defense attorney!

BERISH

There is none—but who is to blame for that? His defenders? He killed them! He massacred His friends and allies! He could have spared Reb Shmuel the dayan, and Reb Yehuda Leib the cantor, and Reb Borukh the teacher, Hersh the sage, and Meilekh the shoemaker! He could have taken care of those who loved Him with all their hearts and believed in Him —in Him alone! Whose fault is it if the earth has become inhabited by assassins—by assassins alone?

MENDEL
By assassins alone? What about us? Our brethren? Are we assassins too?

BERISH
You are clowns, all of you. The earth is inhabited by assassins and clowns.

MENDEL
And Hanna? (*Pause*) And Hanna in all this?

BERISH
Yes, Hanna . . . Hanna, my daughter. I wanted to have the trial on her behalf. You have seen her. She is barely alive; you can't call that living. She sleeps, she sighs, she eats, she listens, she smiles; she is silent: something in her is silent. She speaks silently, she weeps silently; she remembers silently, she screams silently. At times when I look at her I am seized by a mad desire to destroy everything around me. Then I look at her again, closer, and a strange kindness comes over me; I feel like saving the whole world. I am ready to invite all people to come and eat, drink, sing and celebrate—and together drive away the curse that transforms certain people into killers and others into their victims . . . And listen to a clown who makes people laugh. And then, I realize that the clown, that's me.
(*He suddenly regrets having spoken. He shrugs and exits*)

MARIA
You didn't know him before. He was generous and warm toward everybody, Jews and Christians. His wife and I were like sisters. His two sons helped me build the hut for my old mother . . . Why did it have to happen, why?

MENDEL

What happened? *What* happened? Tell us!

MARIA

He has sealed my lips; why open them? Why open old wounds? Can't you imagine what happened? This was a good family, the best. Happiness was deserved and shared. Happiness, happiness . . . (MENDEL *looks at her, pleading with her*) What do you want me to say? We were getting ready to celebrate Hanna's wedding. The best cooks had prepared the best meals. Wine, cake, fruit. Musicians, singers, comedians. Seven holy rabbis had come from faraway villages to participate in the ceremony. Hanna's beauty—how can I describe to you Hanna's divine beauty? Whoever saw her had tears in his eyes—tears of joy and gratitude. Whoever saw her couldn't help but become her friend and protector. There were a hundred guests and more at the inn. Everyone was happy, everyone thanked God for being alive to witness his own happiness. Then . . . *they* arrived. They broke everything. Pillaged all the rooms. Killed the two boys, Hayim and Sholem. Slaughtered all the guests. Beheaded the mistress of the house. And Hanna—they began torturing Hanna. They did things to the poor child. It lasted for hours and hours.

(*She stops*)

MENDEL

Please, Maria, go on.

MARIA

That's all you need to know. That's all there *is* to know.

MENDEL

And the innkeeper?

MARIA

I don't understand.

MENDEL

You told us what happened to Hanna, her brothers and their mother—but not what *they* did to their father.

MARIA

The master fought them with all his strength; he used a hatchet, kitchen knives and clubs; he wounded a few assailants, but he was outnumbered: one against twenty, thirty—more.

MENDEL

Then? What happened then?

MARIA

Nothing.

MENDEL

Go on, Maria! I'm ordering you to continue!

MARIA

I refuse to obey your orders! (*Becomes humble again*) They tied him to the table. Poured wine and alcohol into his throat. And forced him to look.

MENDEL

So he looked. What did he see?

MARIA

I don't know what he saw. Even if I knew, I wouldn't tell you. You have imagination? Use it. Imagine the worst.

MENDEL

I prefer knowing.

MARIA

It's your problem.
(*At this point the door opens. No one notices the* STRANGER. *He listens but does not move forward*)

MENDEL

We want to know, Maria. We must. Perhaps we have been sent here tonight for the sole purpose of learning what happened.

MARIA

You may try, but you'll never succeed. Nobody will. Look here, I was there—and I don't know.

MENDEL

Did you see the innkeeper?

MARIA

Yes, I saw him. I saw what he saw. I cried. I howled like a thousand howling dogs. Not that it mattered. The mob was amused. Excited. The louder I yelled, the more they enjoyed what they were doing.

MENDEL

And the innkeeper?

MARIA

He twistẽd and twisted; he looked and looked, and I shouted and yelled, and the beasts sneered, and little Hanna was covered with blood. Did she know who assaulted her first? And how many followed? It lasted an hour or two, and more, it lasted a whole lifetime, and they left.

MENDEL

You stayed.

MARIA

Of course I did. The priest did too.

MENDEL

The priest?

MARIA

Yes, he came in the middle of the assault.

MENDEL

Didn't he try to stop them?

MARIA

He did. They refused to listen. They were drunk. And busy raping. Pillaging. Murdering. While the beasts were shedding blood, while they ravaged Hanna's body and soul, he lifted his cross—the big one, the one he uses for special occasions—and spoke about love—heavenly love. Nobody listened. They would not have listened to Jesus in person.

MENDEL

And the innkeeper?

MARIA

He kept on staring, staring.

MENDEL

You too?

MARIA

Yes, I stared too. What else could I have done? The beasts kept on raping and exploding with pleasure, the priest kept on drinking and preaching, Hanna kept on suffering more and more pain and shame, the master was shedding tears of blood, and I kept on howling, howling—
(*She stops abruptly;* BERISH *has returned onstage*)

MENDEL
(*To* BERISH)
Now I no longer imagine; now I know.

108

BERISH
You think you know; you don't. You never will.

MENDEL
We stay with you, innkeeper. The trial will be held.

YANKEL
But . . . what about the attorney?

MENDEL
Oh yes, the defense attorney.

AVRÉMEL
Misery of miseries . . . In the whole wide world, from east to west, from south to north, is there no one to plead on behalf of the Almighty? No one to speak for Him?

YANKEL
No one to justify His ways?

AVRÉMEL
No one to sing His glory?

MENDEL
Poor King, poor mankind—one is as much to be pitied as the other . . . In the entire creation, from kingdom to kingdom and nation to nation, is there not one person to be found, one person to take the side of the Creator? Not one believer to explain His mysteries? Not one teacher to love Him in spite of everything, and love Him enough to defend Him against His accusers? Is there no one in the whole universe who would take the case of the Almighty God?

STRANGER
Yes. There is someone. (*Pause*) I will.
(*General commotion. The* STRANGER *smiles.* MARIA *stifles a scream, covering her mouth with both hands*)

MENDEL

Who are you? What do you want?

YANKEL and AVRÉMEL

Who sent you?

STRANGER

I am the one you have been looking for.
  (BERISH *stays close to* MARIA, *as if to defend her*)

MENDEL

The court is in session!

CURTAIN

ACT THREE

Exactly the same as before. Still perturbed, the three judges cannot take their eyes off the STRANGER. *There is something about him that hurts them, almost physically. As for* MARIA, *she seems to withdraw into herself; she is afraid to look at the* STRANGER *or be seen by him.*

MENDEL

Who are you?

STRANGER

My name would mean nothing to you. Call me Sam.

MENDEL

Sam what?

STRANGER

Just Sam.

MENDEL

No family name?

SAM

No family.

MENDEL

No family? Impossible! Surely you have—or had—a father, a mother? Where are they? Where do you come from?

SAM

Must you ask? Must you know? You need a defense attorney and here I am.

BERISH

Have we met before?

SAM

Possibly. I have met many people in many places.

BERISH

Have you been a guest here?

SAM

Possibly. I have been a guest in many homes. You have customers, so do I. Some remember me, others prefer to forget me.

BERISH

I have a strange feeling of having seen you somewhere—here perhaps . . .

YANKEL

Me too. Perhaps in Drohobitz?

SAM

Perhaps.

AVRÉMEL

Perhaps in Amdour?

SAM

Perhaps.

YANKEL

In Kamenetz? Yes, in Kamenetz.

BERISH

Here—

SAM

It's possible. Everything is. I told you: I travel a lot. I meet many people. That's my favorite pastime: to meet people. I like variety. I like to please. To gamble. To win.

MENDEL

What is your occupation?

SAM

Why do you insist on details? Whether I do other things as well, that is my business and, with all due respect, mine alone. If you want another attorney, tell me and I'll be on my way!

MENDEL

No, of course not. Except that we would like to know more about you.

SAM

You all have your little secrets—am I not entitled to mine?
(*The conversation has established a certain rapport between the newcomer and the others. They are willing to accept him. Most of the suspicion has subsided. In a moment they will ask him to play his part. Then, all of a sudden,* MARIA *lets out a scream*)

MARIA

Don't! Don't trust him! Not him! He's mean, evil! Don't let him close! He's Satan himself! I swear it on the life of the Lord! And on my own! He is Satan!
(*All are startled*)

BERISH

I knew it . . . I was right! I knew that my memory wouldn't fool me—

MARIA

Send him away! Good people, I beg you, throw him out before it's too late!

MENDEL

Berish, Maria . . . what are you talking about?

BERISH

I saw him only briefly—a fleeting glimpse—in the darkness, but I was right! Now everything is clear.

MENDEL

What is clear?

MARIA

He has no heart, no soul, no feeling! He's Satan, I'm telling you!

BERISH
(*To* MENDEL)

Don't you understand? They knew each other.

MENDEL

So what? She must have met many customers here.

BERISH

They knew each other intimately.

MENDEL
(*To* SAM)

Did you?

SAM

Indeed we did.

MENDEL

That changes everything. No, it changes nothing. So they knew each other—what's wrong with that? Is that a reason for us to disqualify him? He had an affair. With whom? With a member of the court? No. With the defendant perhaps? No. So what's the problem?

116

MARIA

You don't know. You don't know who he is—what he is,
what he is capable of doing. I know.

MENDEL

Tell us.

MARIA

He is evil. Cruel. He's not human. I'm telling you, he's not
human.

BERISH

It's him, I knew it. I had a glimpse of him just before
. . . before . . .
(MARIA *is hysterical. The* STRANGER *is unmoved, slightly
amused*)

MENDEL

What does this have to do with the trial?

BERISH

I believe Maria.

MENDEL

You are accusing him of what? What happened, Maria? Tell
us. We are your friends.

MARIA

Don't listen to him. Get rid of him. It's bad luck to have him
around.

SAM

Who is on trial here? You decide.

MARIA

Don't listen! Don't listen to him! It's dangerous even to
hear his voice! He perverts the soul and poisons the mind!

MENDEL

But why? Why, Maria?

SAM

Tell them, beautiful Maria. Tell them everything.

MARIA

No! I'm too ashamed!

SAM

You ought to be. But you were not then—were you? (*Pause*)
Can we act like civilized adults? Please tell this hysterical
peasant to keep quiet.

BERISH
(*Jumps at him*)

Now you insult her! You've hurt her, and now you insult
her! I remember now: she cried, she wept, she was not herself.
You destroyed her, and now—

SAM

Innkeeper, innkeeper, you protect her too much. Why do
you protect her so much?

BERISH

You dare to insinuate! One more word, and it'll be your
last!

MENDEL

Please, Berish. Please! He hasn't blamed you for anything
—why get excited over a joke? You were joking, right?

SAM

Always, Your Honor. I'm always joking.

MARIA
(*Contains her tears*)

Don't believe him, don't!

118

MENDEL

If you are not going to tell us everything, you will have to remain silent, Maria.

(MARIA *lets herself fall on the bench, her face in her hands. The* STRANGER *observes her with exaggerated pity*)

SAM

(*To break the mood*)

Let's have another drink, gentlemen. We all need it. Don't worry, innkeeper. I will pay. It's on me.

(SAM *pours drinks. The tension is broken*)

YANKEL

Ah, women! All the same! First they enjoy, then they cry.

AVRÉMEL

I knew some who cried all the time.

YANKEL

Perhaps they enjoyed crying.

AVRÉMEL

I saw them at weddings.

YANKEL

I saw them afterwards—

MENDEL

Enough of this! We are not at the circus!

YANKEL

A pity. A circus has horses.

AVRÉMEL

And bears that dance like people who dance like bears.

YANKEL

Really? I saw only horses; I see horses everywhere.

Also tigers. And lions. And bearded women. And giant dwarfs.

SAM

And judges. And prosecutors. And defendants.

ALL

How dare you? Insolent man!

SAM

Isn't this a circus . . . of sorts?

MENDEL

No. It's theater. There is a difference.

SAM

Really? What is it?

MENDEL

A circus employs only clowns.

SAM

So does the theater.

MENDEL

At the circus you laugh even when you cry.

SAM

At the theater too.

MENDEL

A circus is for children; theater is not.

SAM

I would have preferred to appear at the circus . . . But tonight theater will do.

AVRÉMEL

Can you sing?

SAM

Occasionally I do. But only reluctantly.

AVRÉMEL

How sad.

MENDEL

Who are you?

BERISH

Haven't you heard? He's the stranger who—

MENDEL

—had an affair with—

BERISH

—who was here before—

MENDEL

Who are you when you are not a stranger? (*Pause*) To whom are you not a stranger?

YANKEL

I've seen him somewhere. It must have been in Drohobitz!

AVRÉMEL

Amdour.

MENDEL

All right, we will respect your right to privacy. But do you know what we intend to do here tonight?

SAM

I heard you say a few sentences before; I guessed the rest.

121

MENDEL
Do you know what we expect from you?

SAM
To fulfill my duties as defense attorney.

MENDEL
Do you know on behalf of whom?

SAM
Yes, I do.

MENDEL
And you are not intimidated?

SAM
I am never intimidated.

MENDEL
You are ready to defend your client, just like that, without the slightest hesitation—without any preparation whatsoever? Without asking yourself if perhaps you are not up to what is being demanded of you? (*Pause*) You are not even awed? (*Pause, then louder*) You feel nothing?

SAM
I dislike emotions. I prefer facts and cool logic. As far as I am concerned, we could open the proceedings right now. My client and I are ready.

MENDEL
How about you, Prosecutor?

BERISH
I am ready.

MENDEL
(*Bangs on the table*)
Under the authority vested in us, I open this grave and

solemn trial. We shall listen to the accusation and hear the
defense. And we swear that justice will be done.

SAM

Justice? Whose justice? Yours?

BERISH

What kind of question is that? Justice is justice. Mine, yours,
his: it's the same everywhere. Is there another?

SAM

There is that of God.

BERISH

And it isn't mine? If that is so, then, with your permission
—or without it—I reject it, and for good! I don't want a minor,
secondary justice, a poor man's justice! I want no part of a
justice that escapes me, diminishes me and makes a mockery
out of mine! Justice is here for men and women—I therefore
want it to be human, or let Him keep it!

SAM

You want to reduce God's justice to yours? Why not elevate
yours to His?

MARIA

Look at him! He's talking of justice! The scoundrel, the
dirty scoundrel!

MENDEL

Maria! I forbid you!

BERISH

Let her speak! Why shouldn't the victims of injustice take
part in a debate over justice?

SAM

The prosecutor had better learn the rules and procedures of
the courtroom.

BERISH
Don't tell me what to learn and from whom!

YANKEL
(*Excited*)
Good, very good! Go on, quarrel!

AVRÉMEL
Louder!

YANKEL
Shout! Shout, I'm telling you!

AVRÉMEL
Let your words fight one another!

SAM
My client abhors violence, Your Honor. My client believes
in peace!

BERISH
Ha ha ha! He preaches peace and produces violence!

YANKEL
Good, Berish! Bravo, innkeeper!

AVRÉMEL
How about fighting in rhymes?

BERISH
Are you insane? Are we here to make rhymes?

YANKEL
We're here to celebrate Purim.

AVRÉMEL
And judge the wicked. And reward the just. In rhymes.

124

YANKEL

Purim . . . My horse used to neigh in rhymes, but only on Purim!

AVRÉMEL

Should we wear our masks?

YANKEL

You are a genius.

SAM

Your Honor!
 (*Shows his displeasure*)

MENDEL

I would ask my distinguished colleagues to behave with more dignity! (*Also shows his displeasure*) And Prosecutor, to the point! Please!

SAM

We would deeply appreciate it if the prosecutor would spell out his accusations! What exactly are the charges?

MENDEL
(*To* BERISH)

Prosecutor?

BERISH

I—Berish, Jewish innkeeper at Shamgorod—accuse Him of hostility, cruelty and indifference. Either He dislikes His chosen people or He doesn't care about them—period! But then, why has He chosen us—why not someone else, for a change? Either He knows what's happening to us, or He doesn't wish to know! In both cases He is . . . He is . . . guilty! (*Pause. Loud and clear*) Yes, guilty!
 (*Now the mood has changed. It contains violence.* BERISH *and* SAM *face each other in defiance.* SAM *displays irony;* BERISH, *anger. The court is solemn, uncomfortable*)

125

SAM

Guilty. No less. And you reached that conclusion all by yourself. Let's be serious. You, Prosecutor, are merely a person, whereas my client is—how shall I put it?—more than that. You wish to indict Him? So be it—but then, give us more than anger; give us evidence—that's what counts in a court of law, you know.

BERISH

Evidence? What's that?

SAM

Facts.

BERISH

Facts? What other facts do you want—what other facts do you need? We *are* the facts—we *are* proof, living proof. Look at us! (*Moves closer to him, threatening*) Look at us, and you'll know, and you'll understand. Look well—for we're the only ones you can still see in Shamgorod! The others, all the others are invisible. Absent. Dead. Look at us, I'm telling you, and you'll remember the others!

SAM

I am looking at you, and I see people very much alive, well fed, with no visible marks of poverty. You feed your guests, you offer them lodging—what are you complaining about?

MENDEL

The prosecutor does not complain; he accuses—

SAM

Whom? On what grounds? What does he want?

BERISH

Nothing. I had everything, and everything was taken away from me. But that's besides the point.

126

SAM

What *is* the point?

BERISH

Don't push me: I want the truth to be told.

SAM

Whose truth?

BERISH

Are we starting all over again? Whose truth? Mine! But if mine is not His as well, then He's worse than I thought. Then it would mean that He gave us the taste, the passion of truth without telling us that this truth is not true!

SAM

You wanted Him to tell you everything and do everything for you? He gave you passion—be thankful for that!

BERISH

Thankful! Shame on you and shame on Him for even suggesting that! He gave us suffering, that's what He gave us!

SAM

I know, I know. You have suffered and you are suffering still, and I sympathize, but pain does not constitute judicial evidence.

BERISH

All right. You've got one fact already. Shamgorod. Last year Shamgorod was a village with a Jewish community, a Jewish life. Shamgorod had a Jewish past and a Jewish future. Jewish warmth and Jewish songs could be found here in every street, in every house. Go look for them now. Shamgorod is mute. Its silence—what is it if not a fact? Three houses of study —demolished, pillaged; the main synagogue—burned down; the sacred scrolls—profaned. Aren't the ruins facts? Aren't the ashes glowing with facts? Over a hundred Jewish families lived here; now there is one—and this one is mutilated, maimed,

deprived of joy and hope. What is all this to you—and Him?
(*He raises his hand, as if ready to strike the adversary*) What is this,
I'm asking you?

SAM

Sad.

BERISH

What did you say?

SAM

Sad. It is sad.

MENDEL

Is that *all* you have to say?

SAM

Oh, I do not dispute the events, but I consider them to be
highly irrelevent to the case before us, Your Honor. I do not
deny that blood was shed and that life was extinguished, but
I am asking the question: Who is to blame for all that? After
all, the situation seems to me simple indeed: men and women
and children were massacred by other men. Why involve, why
implicate their Father in Heaven?

BERISH

You want to leave Him out? Turn Him into a neutral by-
stander? Would a father stand by quietly, silently, and watch
his children being slaughtered?

SAM

By whom? By his other children!

BERISH

All right, by his other children! Would he not interfere?
Should he not?

SAM

You are using images, let me add mine. When human be-

128

ings kill one another, where is God to be found? You see Him among the killers. I find Him among the victims.

BERISH

He—a victim? A victim is powerless; is He powerless? He is almighty, isn't He? He could use His might to save the victims, but He doesn't! So—on whose side is He? Could the killer kill without His blessing—without His complicity?

SAM

Are you suggesting that the Almighty is on the side of the killer?

BERISH

He is not on the side of the victim.

SAM

How do you know? Who told you?

BERISH

The killers told me. They told the victims. They always do. They always say loud and clear that they kill in the name of God.

SAM

Did the victims tell you? (BERISH *hesitates*) No? Then how do you know? Since when do you take the killers' word for granted? Since when do you place your faith in them? They are efficient killers but poor witnesses.

BERISH

You would like to hear the victims? So would I. But they do not talk. They cannot come to the witness stand. They're dead. You hear me? The witnesses for the prosecution are the dead. All of them. I could call them, summon them a thousand times, and they would not appear here before you. They are not accustomed to taking a walk outside, and surely not on Purim eve. You want to know where they are? At the cemetery. At the bottom of mass graves. I implore the court to consider their absence as the weightiest of proofs, as the heaviest of accusations. They are witnesses, Your Honor, invisible and silent witnesses, but still witnesses! Let their testimony enter your conscience and your memory! Let their premature, unjust deaths turn into an outcry so forceful that it will make the universe tremble with fear and remorse!

SAM

Too easy, Your Honor. What gives the prosecutor the right to speak for the dead?

BERISH

I knew them alive. I witnessed their death.

SAM

So what? Does he know, is he empowered to know what they felt and thought and believed when they died? He depicts them as accusers—or witnesses for the prosecution. What if they felt differently? Suppose they chose, at that supreme hour, to repent! Suppose they were pleased—yes, pleased—to leave this ugly planet behind them and enter a world of eternal peace and truth?

BERISH

That's too much! Even for him! (*To* SAM) You really believe that people want to die, love to die? That they are happy to die? Either you're crazy or cynical! Woe to God if you're His defender!

SAM

I would like the court to remind the prosecution of its obligation not to indulge in personal attacks and insults! Does he wish to see me dismissed?

BERISH

But *he* is insulting the dead!

SAM

Why is that an insult? I would go one step further and say

that they departed from this world uttering words of gratitude—

BERISH

For what? For being slaughtered?

SAM

—for dying without prolonged suffering or shame. There are a thousand ways in which men die, you know.

BERISH

A lie, it's a lie! There are a thousand ways to suffer, but only one way to die—and death is always cruel, unjust, inhuman.

SAM

No, my dear Prosecutor. In these matters I am a greater expert than you. There are moments of death more cruel than others.

BERISH

You're telling me? More cruel, yes! Less cruel, no! (*To the court*) Take Reb Hayim the scribe, who never squashed a fly or an ant, for they too are God's living creatures; I saw him in agony. I want to know: Who willed his agony? Take Shmuel the cobbler, who treated strangers as though they were his own children; I saw his tears, his last tears. I demand an answer: Who was thirsty for his blood? I want to know: Why was Reb Yiddel the cantor murdered? or Reb Monish his brother? Why were Hava the orphan and her little brother Zisha murdered? So that they could say thank you—and I could say thank you?

SAM

Again you speak for them? You act as though they had appointed you their spokesman. Have they? You knew them —so what? Alive, they were yours; dead, they belong to someone else. The dead belong to the dead, and together they form an immense community reposing in God and loving Him the way you have never loved and never will! (*To the court*) He is asking, Why murder—why death? Pertinent questions. But we have some more: Why evil—why ugliness? If God chooses not to answer, He must have his reasons. God is God, and His will is independent from ours—as is His reasoning.

MENDEL

What is there left for us to do?

SAM

Endure. Accept. And say Amen.

BERISH

Never! If He wants my life, let Him take it. But He has taken other lives—Don't tell me they were happy to submit to His will—don't tell me they're happy now! If I'm not, and I'm alive, how can they be? True, they are silent. Good for them and good for Him. If they choose to be silent, that's their business! I shall not be!

SAM

That is understandable. They saw His charity and grace; you did not.

BERISH

Maria, you are right. He *is* repulsive. (*To* SAM) How can you speak of grace and charity after a pogrom?

SAM

Is there a more propitious time to speak about them? You are alive—isn't that a proof of His kindness?

BERISH

The Jews of Shamgorod perished—isn't that a proof of His lack of kindness?

SAM

You are obsessed with the dead; I only think of the living.

BERISH

And what if I told you that He spared me not out of kindness but out of cruelty?

SAM

He spared you, and you are against Him.

BERISH

He annihilated Shamgorod and you want me to be for Him? I can't! If He insists upon going on with His methods, let Him —but I won't say Amen. Let Him crush me, I won't say Kaddish. Let Him kill me, let Him kill us all, I shall shout and shout that it's His fault. I'll use my last energy to make my protest known. Whether I live or die, I submit to Him no longer.

SAM

He spared you, and you anger Him. He spared you, and you hurt Him, you make Him suffer.

BERISH

Don't talk to me of His suffering—leave that to the priest. If I am given the choice of feeling sorry for Him or for human beings, I choose the latter anytime. He is big enough, strong enough to take care of Himself; man is not.

SAM

(*With some warmth*)

What do you know of God that enables you to denounce Him? You turn your back on Him—then you describe Him! Why? Because you witnessed a pogrom? Think of our ancestors, who, throughout centuries, mourned over the massacre of their beloved ones and the ruin of their homes—and yet they repeated again and again that God's ways are just. Are we worthier than they were? Wiser? Purer? Are we more pious than the rabbis of York, the students of Magenza? More privileged than the dreamers of Saloniki, the Just of Prague and Drohobitz? Do we possess more rights than they did over heaven or truth? After the destruction of the Temple of Jerusa-

133

lem, our forefathers wept and proclaimed *umipnei khataenou*—
it's all because of our sins. Their descendants said the same
thing during the Crusades. And the Holy Wars. The same
thing during the pogroms. And now you want to say something else? Does the massacre of Shamgorod weigh more than
the burning of the Sanctuary? Is the ruin of your homes a more
heinous crime than the ransacking of God's city? Does the
death of your community imply a greater meaning than the
disappearance of the communities of Zhitomir, Nemirov,
Tlusk and Berditchev? Who are you to make comparisons or
draw conclusions? Born in dust, you are nothing but dust.

BERISH

If He wanted me to be dust, why hasn't He left me as dust?
But I'm not dust. I'm standing up, I'm walking, thinking,
wondering, shouting: I'm human!

SAM

So were our ancestors.

BERISH

And they kept quiet? Too bad—then I'll speak for them,
too. For them, too, I'll demand justice. For the widows of
Jerusalem and the orphans of Betar. For the slaves of Rome
and Capadoccia. And for the destitute of Oman and the victims of Koretz. I'll shout for them, against Him I'll shout. To
you, judges, I'll shout, "Tell Him what He should not have
done; tell Him to stop the bloodshed now. Discharge your
duties without fear!"

MENDEL

We shall discharge our duties, innkeeper, but it will not be
without fear.

SAM

Duties, duties . . . what big words . . . Your duties as what?
As judges or as Jews?

134

MENDEL

Are the two incompatible?

SAM

The judges judge; Jews are being judged.

MENDEL

By whom?

SAM

First by God, then by other nations. We are in exile, you know.

BERISH

In exile, yet free! Members of the court, answer me: Are you free? I know it's all a game—it's theater; but within this game, are you free? Do you act the part of free men? Answer me!

(*He is staring at the three judges with such anxiety that they are unable to reply; it takes them a minute to take hold of themselves*)

MENDEL

Tonight we are all free.

SAM

(*Laughs disquietingly*)

In some communities there is a custom of crowning a fool King of Purim. He is given a queen. Their kingdom lasts but one day, one night.

MENDEL

One night will be enough; it will be more than nothing— the opposite of nothing.

SAM

You are free—and what are you going to do with your freedom?

MENDEL

We shall be free—we shall judge freely—that will be all.

SAM

Will you judge without preconceived ideas?

MENDEL

Yes.

SAM

Without prejudice?

MENDEL

Yes.

SAM

Without passion?

MENDEL

No. With passion.

SAM

The verdict will be worthless!

MENDEL

It may be worthless, but it will be handed down nevertheless.

MARIA
(*Rises*)

Even if you have a living witness? (*Pause*) If you have an eyewitness, will the verdict still be worthless?

MENDEL

Aren't you the audience? You have no right to intervene in the debate.

136

MARIA

I changed my mind. I want to testify.
(*She moves forward to face the court. As witness, she seems
more determined, almost vengeful*)

MENDEL

Why, Maria? Why did you change your part—and your
mind?

MARIA

You need a witness? Here I am. I have seen everything. I
can testify, I have the right to. The duty as well.

SAM

I am not sure.

MENDEL

What do you mean? Why should her testimony not be
accepted?

SAM

Well . . . she is not even Jewish.

BERISH

Are you? And even if you are, what difference does it make?
Since when may witnesses be disqualified because of their
religion? They must be honest—that's all. And I, Berish, the
innkeeper of Shamgorod, vouch for her honesty.

MENDEL

Do you swear that you will tell the truth and nothing but
the truth?

MARIA

Of course I do. But not the whole truth. The whole truth
cannot be told—and yet I know the truth.

SAM

We have a Purim court—now we have a Purim witness!

137

MENDEL

You are intimidating the witness!

SAM

Listen, Your Honor, I was not going to tell you—I did not want to embarrass her in public, but since you insist . . . She is not what one might call an honorable woman. I would even go a step further and say that she is not what one might call a respectable woman.

BERISH

(*With hardly contained violence*)

You dirty swine!

SAM

No, not me; she is dirty. I wasn't going to say aloud what people say in whispers, but this is a court of law. The truth must be told.

BERISH

I'll strangle you with my own hands!

MARIA

(*To* BERISH)

Let him speak. (*She bites her lips*) Yes, Berish. I want to hear him speak.

BERISH

What for? I can do without his lies.

MARIA

So can I. Still, I want to hear them.

SAM

Lies? Must they be lies? Are you sure they will be? Members of the court, I owe you the truth: I have known this woman.

MENDEL

That much we guessed.

SAM

With the court's permission, I would like to explain the circumstances of our meeting—no, of our involvement. I came to spend the night here. I paid for space above the stove. I was alone. Not for long, though. I was half awake when I felt someone looking at me in the dark. Then she lay down next to me. Next to me? No, close to me. Closer. I could hardly understand what was happening when she began doing what honorable and respectable women must never do. She seduced me, members of the court. I resisted, I swear I did, but she knows how to get to men and weaken their resolve. She has had experience . . . And you were ready to receive her testimony!

BERISH

Dirty, dirty swine! I'll break your bones! Just wait!

SAM

I understand your anger—I would not have believed either that this woman could be so indecent and lack so much . . . restraint.

BERISH
(*Ready to attack him*)

Stop it!

SAM

Do you think I am inventing this?

BERISH

What do I think? That you're lying, that's what I think.

SAM

I am not, innkeeper. She and I—we spent a long night together. You do not believe me? Ask her. (*To* MARIA) Did we spend a long, delightful night together, yes or no?
    (MARIA *is transfixed. It is as though she could not believe her own ears*)

MARIA
(*Still staring at* SAM)
Yes.

SAM
Near the stove?

MARIA
Yes.

SAM
Did you feel . . . pleasure?

MARIA
I did.

SAM
(*To* BERISH)
Well?

BERISH
You used force!

SAM
(*To* MARIA)
Did I?

MARIA
No.

BERISH
Don't tell me you charmed her! You used sorcery . . .

SAM
Ask her.

MARIA
He did. I knew much happiness with him—I would never
have guessed so much happiness existed.

(SAM *shrugs off* BERISH *'s outbursts. All eyes are on* MARIA. *Transformed. Tender as never before. Is she dreaming?*)

MARIA

Evil—is there no limit to evil? It's like pain. So much pain then, and yet some was left for now. I don't understand why . . . Walks in the field. Whispers. Silences. Timid caresses. He spoke of his love for me. He couldn't live without me. It was the first time anyone spoke to me like that. "But I've just met you," I said. Yes, but he'd seen me. Many times. From far, far away. A relative's house, a friend's farm. But— no but. I ran, he ran after me. I refused to listen, I heard nevertheless. "That's love," he said. It was the first time I believed it is possible to be madly in love. Words, more words. More meetings at night. Words—I began waiting for them. My life was empty, empty of certain words. His made my blood run faster. Set my mind on fire. . . . Words became caresses. I was confused. Disturbed. Couldn't think or see. "Love," he kept on saying. "Love justifies everything." I was afraid of the word "everything"; also of the word "love." But— no but. One evening I ran away from him. To my room. And forgot to lock the door.

SAM

(*Sneers*)

How convenient . . .

MARIA

He opened it. Said he couldn't live without me. Cried and laughed. Threatened and promised. All the while whispering, whispering that love is more precious than life itself . . . His hands. His face. His lips. On me. In me. A scream. His? Mine? I thought, Love, that's what they call love. (*Long pause. No one, not even* SAM, *dares interrupt her recollection*) Then . . . the awakening. The change. He stood up and hit me in the face. With anger. And hate. "You cheap harlot," he shouted. "You fell for it, you really did!" More blows and more words: which hurt more? They kept raining on me. I was impure, unworthy because I let him seduce me. He spat on me. What do they

call that? I wondered. I didn't know then; now I do. Evil.
That's what they call evil.

(*She has spoken without hatred, without passion; only with
sadness. And amazement.* SAM *feels he must say something
to counteract the effect of her statement*)

SAM

And you believe her? How gullible you are! She says she
resisted for many nights. Why didn't Berish see me with her
then?

BERISH

I did!

SAM

How many times?

BERISH

Once . . . I remember it well because it was just before
. . . before—

SAM

She says that I came more than once to pursue her. Really,
can you see me pursue . . . her? Furthermore, if we had time,
I would prove to you that I could not have been here more
than once: when she says she saw me here, I was visiting
friends elsewhere . . . in Marozka. Yes, the small town where
our brethren were killed. I am saying this not to justify myself
—I am not on trial, am I?—but to show why this woman is
disqualified as a witness . . . But she is not the only one we
have!

MENDEL

She is not? What do you mean?

SAM

She is young and beautiful.

142

BERISH

You'll die first! You won't live to set your dirty eyes on her!
(*Commotion.* BERISH *is more violent than ever.* SAM *is using the question as diversion:* MARIA*'s testimony is now forgotten*)

MENDEL

Hanna is ill. We saw her earlier. She must not be disturbed.

SAM

We are not going to hurt her, are we? We will ask her a few
questions and send her back to bed. What is wrong with that?

BERISH

I'll tell you what's wrong. She's my daughter, not yours. She
has seen enough criminals; I don't want her to see you, too.

SAM

Members of the court! There is one eyewitness *and* victim
in this house. Isn't it our sacred duty to listen to her testimony?
(*The three judges exchange whispers*)

MENDEL

I don't understand you, Defense Attorney. Supposing we
decide to summon her to the stand, surely she would help the
prosecution, not the defense.

SAM

My client and I beg to differ, Your Honor. In our view,
witnesses serve neither the prosecution nor the defense; they
serve truth and truth alone.

BERISH

You're not going to get my daughter!

SAM

Your daughter is of no interest to this court; the witness is.

143

BERISH
You're not going to get her!

SAM
What are you afraid of? Are we not a group of respectable and honorable men—charitable, too—who would actually like nothing better than to help her and comfort her! Really, innkeeper!

BERISH
You're not going to get her!

YANKEL
Actually—

BERISH
You're not going—

AVRÉMEL
You *are* afraid!

BERISH
She is. Afraid of all men. You're not going to—

AVREMEL
Don't you trust *us*? She has seen us; she was not afraid of us.

YANKEL
(*Reassuringly*)
She will be under our protection, innkeeper. Do not worry.

AVRÉMEL
Please. Trust us. It will not last long. A minute. Please, go.

YANKEL
We would be honored to see her again.

BERISH
(*To* SAM)
You'll pay for this . . .
(*Exits, followed by* MARIA)

YANKEL
I used to like Purim.

AVRÉMEL
I loved all holidays.

MENDEL
I did not. I don't like to be told when to rejoice.

YANKEL
I do.

MENDEL
You can force yourself to accept sadness, not joy.

SAM
Is there a difference?

MENDEL
Oh, there is, Stranger, there is. (*Pause*) Haven't we two met before? (*Pause*) Have you ever been in Zhironov? (*Pause*) Have you ever heard of Zhironov?
(SAM *answers none of the questions. To break the uneasy mood,* YANKEL *speaks*)

YANKEL
I have.

AVRÉMEL
The famous massacre of Zhironov. All the Jews perished there.

MENDEL
All—except one.

145

YANKEL

You never told us—

AVRÉMEL

You came to us from Zhironov?

YANKEL

Were you there when—

MENDEL

Yes. I was there.

AVRÉMEL

How did you manage to escape?

SAM

There is always one singled out to escape.

YANKEL

A miracle!

SAM

There is always someone to call it a miracle.

MENDEL
(*To* SAM)

Were you there—then? No, you couldn't have been. Perhaps before? I seem to remember you in Zhironov . . .
(*Again,* SAM *does not answer. Again,* YANKEL *breaks the silence*)

YANKEL

What happened? How—

MENDEL

Sabbath morning. A crowded synagogue—more crowded than usual. I stood on the bimah before the open scrolls and read. That Shabbat we read the commandment to celebrate our holidays in joy. I had hardly finished the sentence when

146

the doors were pushed open. The mob took over. The killers were laughing. I remember their laughter as I remember their shiny swords. Minutes later, it was all over. Not one Jew cried out; we didn't have the time. As I heard the echo of my own words: "And you shall celebrate your holidays in joy"—I found myself without a community. I was still standing; I stood throughout the slaughter. Standing before the open parchments. Why was I spared? Is it possible that they failed to see me because I was standing? I saw blood, only blood. I felt swept by madness. I whispered over and over again: "And you shall celebrate your holidays in joy, in joy, in joy." And I backed out and left.

SAM

Blessed be the Lord for His miracles.

MENDEL

A whole community was massacred, and you talk of miracles?

SAM

A Jew survived, and you ignore them?

AVRÉMEL

The mob was struck blind. How was it possible?

SAM

Miracles are miracles; they don't call for explanations.

YANKEL

They happen; they should happen more often.
    (HANNA, *in white, enters, escorted by* BERISH *and* MARIA)

MARIA

Do not be afraid, sweet little girl, do not be afraid.

HANNA

Why should I be afraid? Have you ever seen me afraid?

MARIA

No, sweet Hanna. Of course not.

HANNA

Do you know why? To show fear is to believe in misfortune.
Well, I don't.

MARIA

Of course, sweet soul. Nothing will happen. Surely not
tonight.

HANNA

Not tonight?

MARIA

Tonight is Purim.

HANNA

I wish I could play the part of Queen Esther. May I?

MARIA

Anything, sweet little Hanna. You may play anything you
wish. You may do anything you desire. We are here.

HANNA

Is she happy?

MARIA

Who?

HANNA

Esther. Queen Esther. Is she happy?

MENDEL

She must be. She is beautiful, rich, powerful; she gets what
she wants. From everybody.

HANNA

A pity.

148

MENDEL

A pity? Why a pity?

HANNA

I will not be able to play Queen Esther. But then, perhaps she is not happy; she only pretends.

SAM

Quite possible, young lady. I admire your charm as well as your intelligence. What you just said is possible if not probable: Esther is not happy, because she is being lied to. Everybody lies to her. The old king, her uncle, her friends. But not Haman: he doesn't lie. They all used her; not he. That makes her even more unhappy.

HANNA

Ah yes, Haman! If I play Esther, will you be Haman?

SAM

At your service, Majesty.

HANNA

Who is the king? (*To* MENDEL) You? Yes, you. And my uncle Mordechai? (*To* YANKEL) You?

YANKEL

What does he have to do?

HANNA

Be sad.

YANKEL
(*Pointing to* AVRÉMEL)

Let him be sad!

HANNA

And where are my brothers and sisters? Those that need me? Those whom I must save? Where are they? I want to see them! Their children with their innocent voices . . . their old

men with their words of wisdom . . . their brides, their grooms
. . . Where are they? Dead? Esther has not saved them. No
one has. Poor queen. Again, she was lied to.

YANKEL

But it's not in the book.

SAM

Then it's in another book.

HANNA

I don't like you.

SAM

Naturally—I am Haman. Haman does not lie. And he will
tell you something that no one is willing to admit: it's all the
queen's fault. The persecutions, the suffering, the anguish—
it's all because of her. She must have sinned many times, with
many men, to have caused such pain and so much desolation.

HANNA

But I hear music. Laughter. Shouts of happiness. I hear a
father and a mother wishing each other *mazel tov.* I hear a
voice, mine perhaps, yelling, "Arye-Leib, Arye-Leib . . ."

MENDEL

Poor Queen Esther. She remembers Hanna.

YANKEL

I want to become a judge again.

HANNA

"Arye-Leib," a voice is crying "Arye-Leib." He does not
hear, he cannot, he is dead. I am dead.

YANKEL

I demand to become a judge again!

HANNA

The queen is dead, and yet it is the most beautiful day in
her life. Remember, Maria?

(HANNA *seems happy*)

BERISH

She remembers, and so do I. And I would give all that I
have, my life included, to make her forget . . . They killed
Arye-Leib. And his old father. And the witnesses to the wedding. And the rabbis who were about to perform the ceremony. And the musicians. The guests. They killed and killed
. . . and I remember, I remember . . .

MENDEL

Go on, innkeeper. Shamgorod, Drohobitz, Zhironov, they
are all alike. We must tell the tale, we must remember. Tell
us everything. We shall remember.

BERISH

You have heard enough. But not all.

AVRÉMEL

I listen to you, innkeeper, and I imagine Purim without the
miracle of Purim. And I know everything.

BERISH

Imagine the Jews of Shushan—and Shamgorod—mutilated,
knifed, disfigured, thrown into the street, into the mud. Imagine their Queen Esther—so sweet and trusting, pure and radi-
ant—imagine her covered with blood and dirt, imagine her
lying on the floor with drunkards waiting in line . . . Can you
imagine?

MENDEL

I do not have to imagine; I *know.*

MARIA

Come, Hanna. Let us go back to your room.

HANNA
Arye-Leib, I am so happy, Arye-Leib. We are immortal.
And rich. The forest is ours. The rivers. The stars—they shine
brighter. And life is calling us, as we call life. Nothing frightens us, nothing leaves us indifferent; we live at the center of
the world; we are the center of the world.

MARIA
(*To the court*)
We are playing theater; but you make her suffer, and her
suffering is real.

MENDEL
It's a *Purimschpiel,* Maria. You are right. Take Hanna back
to her room.

HANNA
A *Purimschpiel* . . . When Purim is over, the actors remove
their masks, don't they? The dead get up and the living start
laughing again. When is Purim over?
(MARIA *leads her to the door and they meet the* PRIEST, *who
has been standing there; he has heard* HANNA's *question*)

PRIEST
Soon, Hanna. Purim will be over very soon.

MARIA
You again?

PRIEST
I cannot sleep, Maria. This time it's not because of you.
(*To the others*) Am I disturbing you again?

SAM
You never disturb us.

MARIA
Only on Purim. Except that whenever you come, it's always
Purim.

PRIEST

I cannot sleep. I tried . . . Like the old king of your book, what's his name, I had bad dreams. So I decided to come back to my friend Berish and his guests.

MENDEL

You did the right thing. (*Has an idea*) Any news? Have you learned anything?

PRIEST

It's late, later than I thought. (*To* BERISH) You've refused to listen. You should have taken your daughter and your friends and fled as far away as possible. Now it's too late.

BERISH
(*With irony*)

Except, of course, if we kiss your cross—right?

PRIEST

Do not make fun of me, friend. The cross itself would no longer protect you: the killers respect it less than you do. But we could try . . .

MENDEL

Why did you come back now?

PRIEST

I don't know. To help you, of course.

MENDEL

What do you think we should do?

PRIEST

I don't know. They are too close. They are watching the inn. They are everywhere.

YANKEL

Another pogrom?

AVREMEL

Another trial.

MENDEL

What can we do?

PRIEST

I don't know, I'm telling you. What I do know is that whatever you do, you must do it now.

BERISH

What you mean is—I know what you mean. Well, the answer is no. My sons and my fathers perished without betraying their faith; I can do no less.

SAM

My dear, dear Prosecutor, you baffle me. You speak of faith, of sacrifice, of martyrdom. Have you forgotten the trial? What you said about my client?

PRIEST

What . . . what's that?

BERISH

(*To* SAM)

This has nothing to do with you or your client. (*Pause*) It's a personal decision.

PRIEST

Berish, my friend Berish. You are all drunk, so am I—perhaps. But I beg you: let's do something while there is still time! (*Pause. He decides to have courage*) Why can't you try—I say try—my solution temporarily? Nobody will ever know anything about it, I swear to you. (*Has a better idea*) You know what? Let's do it in the spirit of your Purim holiday. As a farce. With masks. You do me a favor, and perhaps—I say perhaps —you will stay alive; I'll handle the mob. And tomorrow,

when Purim is over, you remove the masks—and become Jewish again. Well? What do you think, innkeeper?
(*The three judges are flabbergasted.* HANNA *smiles*)

BERISH

I said what I had to say. My answer is no. Ask the others. Maybe you'll have better luck with them.
(*The* PRIEST *turns to the others. The three judges shake their heads*)

SAM

Thank you, Priest. Your concern touches us deeply. We are not going to accept your solution—we all have our reasons. Anyway, you said it yourself: the killers respect nothing.

PRIEST

So there is nothing for me to do?

MENDEL

There is something. Go to the village. Try to alert some of your better and wiser parishioners. Get in touch with the authorities. They may still arrive in time. Miracles are always possible.
(*The* PRIEST *is sad. He looks at all the characters. Tears well up in his eyes. He wants to shake* BERISH's *hand but decides against it; will they meet again? No. But why admit it publicly? He leaves without saying a word*)

YANKEL

Is there a cellar?

AVRÉMEL

An underground passage?

MARIA

Yes, there is a cellar.

YANKEL

There must be an attic.

AVRÉMEL

How about making a run for it? It's still dark.

MENDEL

And the trial? The verdict?

SAM

I take note of the important fact that the prosecutor opted
for God against the enemy of God; he did so at the sacrifice
of his life. Does it mean that the case is to be dismissed?

BERISH

Not at all! I have not opted for God. I'm against His enemies, that's all.

MENDEL

So—it is going to start all over again. Jews and their enemies
will face one another once more. And then? Purim will be
over. Who will continue the thread of our tale? The last page
will not be written. But the one before? It is up to us to
prepare testimony for future generations. Thus I am asking
you for the last time: What about the trial? The verdict?

BERISH

As far as I'm concerned, the trial will go on. I haven't
changed; I'm not going to change now.

MENDEL

The end is near, and you refuse to forgive?

BERISH

I lived as a Jew, and it is as a Jew that I shall die—and it is
as a Jew that, with my last breath, I shall shout my protest to
God! And because the end is near, I shall shout louder! Because the end is near, I'll tell Him that He's more guilty than
ever!

(MENDEL *smiles and turns to the defense attorney for his
final remarks*)

156

SAM

First of all, I wish to pay tribute to the loyalty and courage of my distinguished colleague and opponent. The fact that he refused to give up his faith does him—and us—honor. As for his stubborn attitude with regard to the Almighty, of course I cannot but disagree. I understand him, but I disapprove. God is just, and His ways are just.

MENDEL

Even now?

SAM

Now and forever.

MENDEL

Just? How can anyone proclaim Him just—now? With the end so near? Look at us, look at Hanna, search your own memory: between Jews who suffer and die, and God who does not—how can you choose God?

SAM

I must. I'm His servant. He created the world and me without asking for my opinion; He may do with both whatever He wishes. Our task is to glorify Him, to praise Him, to love Him—in spite of ourselves.

MENDEL

But how *can* you?

SAM

It's simple. Faith in God must be as boundless as God Himself. If it exists at the expense of man, too bad. God is eternal, man is not.

MENDEL
(*Moves closer to him*)

Who are you, Stranger?

SAM

I told you. I am God's defender.

MENDEL

Who are you when you are not performing? When you are
not defending Him?

SAM

Why do you want to know?

MENDEL

Because I envy you. Your love of God: I wish I had one
measure of it. Your piety: I wish it were mine. Your faith:
mine is less profound, less intact than yours. Who are you?

SAM

I am not allowed to reveal myself to you. (*In a low voice*) And
what if I told you that I am God's emissary? I visit His creation
and bring stories back to Him. I see all things, I watch all men.
I cannot do all I want, but I can undo all things. Have I said
enough?

MENDEL

Enough for me to envy you even more. Throughout the
proceedings, you have demonstrated a respect for God that I
find admirable. And yet, we know already that God is to be
loved but also feared. In truth, if I had to pronounce a verdict
right now, it would be, I think, influenced by Berish the
innkeeper . . . But we are not going to have enough time for
our deliberations. The verdict will be announced by someone
else, at a later stage. For the trial will continue—without us.
Still, I wish I knew who you are. To follow your example.

MARIA
(*Whispering*)
You're crazy, you're all crazy . . .

MENDEL
After all, let's be frank: in the whole wide world of sorrow
and agony, there was only one man, one alone, who chose to
defend the honor and the glory, the justice and the kindness
of God—and that was you. Who are you, Stranger? A saint?
A penitent? A prophet in disguise?

MARIA
Crazy, I'm telling you . . . We're all crazy . . .

YANKEL
(*Infected by* MENDEL's *fervor*)
A wonder rabbi?

AVRÉMEL
A miracle maker?

YANKEL
An emissary sent from the kingdom of the Ten Lost Tribes?

AVRÉMEL
A mystical dreamer on his way to meet—and make us meet
—the Redeemer?

YANKEL
Is this why you . . . played with Maria?

AVRÉMEL
Yes, yes: you took her so as to penetrate the depth of sin
and lift up its holy sparks.
(*The door opens. The* PRIEST *reappears. From his expression,
we understand: everything is lost. In the other doorway*
HANNA *stands*)

BERISH
This time I'll kill. I swear to you: I'll kill.
(*They all begin building defense positions. Pushing tables to
the doors. They barricade the windows.* BERISH *prepares long*

159

knives and hatchets. Suddenly there is collective hysteria. They
all gather around SAM *and beg him to save them*)

YANKEL
(*To* SAM)
You *are* a hidden Just; intercede on our behalf!

AVRÉMEL
You are a messenger; do something!

MENDEL
You are close to heaven, pray for us! Your faith must be
rewarded! Invoke it!

BERISH
I'll kill, I'll kill . . .

YANKEL
Say Psalms, holy man!

AVRÉMEL
Order the angels to come to our rescue!

YANKEL
You must accomplish miracles, you can! We know you can!
Please!

AVRÉMEL
Think of Hanna—save her! Think of us—save us!

MENDEL
You are a *tzaddik,* a Just, a Rabbi, a Master—you are en-
dowed with mystical powers; you are a holy man. Do something to revoke the decree! If you cannot, who could? You are
God's only defender, you have rights and privileges: use
them! For heaven's sake, use them! Oh holy man, we beg you
to save God's children from further shame and suffering!
(*All candles, save one, are put out. Strange sounds are heard*
outside. SAM *walks from one person to another, smiling reas-*

suringly. Then he stops before MENDEL *and scrutinizes him*)

YANKEL

It's Purim. Let's wear our masks!
(*The three judges put theirs on.* SAM *pulls his out of his pocket and raises it to his face. All shout in fear, and Satan speaks to them, laughing*)

SAM

So—you took me for a saint, a Just? Me? How could you be that blind? How could you be that stupid? If you only knew, if you only knew . . .
(*Satan is laughing. He lifts his arm as if to give a signal. At that precise moment the last candle goes out, and the door opens, accompanied by deafening and murderous roars*)

CURTAIN

BOOKS BY ELIE WIESEL

Available from Schocken

A BEGGAR IN JERUSALEM

In the days following the Six-Day War, a Holocaust survivor visits the reunited city of Jerusalem. At the Western Wall he encounters the beggars and madmen who congregate there every evening, and who force him to confront the ghosts of his past and his ties to the present.

THE GATES OF THE FOREST

A young Jew hiding from the Nazis in the forests and small towns of Eastern Europe allows another refugee to sacrifice himself in his stead. As he struggles with his guilt, one question recurs: How to live in a world that God has abandoned?

LEGENDS OF OUR TIME

From a rabbi at Auschwitz who fasts on Yom Kippur, to a young Spanish Catholic whose discovery of an ancient Marrano document starts him on a quest to regain his lost heritage, Wiesel's encounters with fifteen extraordinary men and women resonate with the poetry and passion of Jewish spiritual resistance.

THE TOWN BEYOND THE WALL

Based on Wiesel's own life, this is the story of a young Holocaust survivor who returns to his hometown after the liberation, seeking to understand the mystery of what he calls "the face in the window"—the symbol of all those who just stood by and watched as innocent men, women, and children were led to the slaughter.

THE TRIAL OF GOD

When three itinerant actors arrive in a small Eastern European village to perform a Purim play for the Jewish community, they are horrified to discover that all but two of the Jewish residents have been murdered in a recent pogrom. The actors decide to stage a mock trial of God, indicting Him for allowing such things to happen to His children.

Available from Vintage

A JEW TODAY

In this powerful collection of essays, letters, and diary entries, Wiesel probes such central moral and political issues as Zionism and the Middle East conflict, anti-Semitism in the former U.S.S.R., the obligations of American Jews toward Israel, and the media's treatment of the Holocaust.

AVAILABLE AT YOUR LOCAL BOOKSTORE *or*
To order by mail, please fill out or copy the form below and send to:
Random House Order Department,
400 Hahn Road, Westminster, Maryland 21157.
To order by phone, call 1-800-733-3000 (credit cards only).

- If you wish to pay by check or money order, please make it payable to Random House, Inc.
- If you prefer to charge your order to a major credit card, please fill in the information below.

Charge my account with

❏ American Express   ❏ Visa   ❏ MasterCard

Account No. _____ Expiration Date _____

(Signature) _____

Name _____

Address _____

City/State/Zip _____

TITLE	ISBN	QUANTITY	PRICE	TOTAL
A Beggar in Jerusalem	0-8052-0897-6	_____ x	$14.00	= _____
The Gates of the Forest	0-8052-0896-8	_____ x	$13.00	= _____
A Jew Today	0-394-74057-2	_____ x	$ 9.00	= _____
Legends of Our Time	0-8052-0714-7	_____ x	$14.00	= _____
The Town Beyond the Wall	0-8052-0697-3	_____ x	$13.00	= _____
The Trial of God	0-8052-0809-7	_____ x	$12.00	= _____

Shipping/Handling* = _____

Subtotal = _____

Sales Tax (where applicable) = _____

Total Enclosed = $_____

*In addition to the price of the books, enclose shipping and handling: $2.00 for the first book and $0.50 for each additional book ordered.
Prices subject to change without notice. Please allow 4-6 weeks for delivery.